大腸癌取扱い規約（英語版 第3版）
［大腸癌取扱い規約 第9版 準拠］

Japanese Classification of Colorectal, Appendiceal, and Anal Carcinoma

 Japanese Society for Cancer of the Colon and Rectum

Third English Edition

Kanehara & Co., Ltd.

ISBN 978-4-307-20395-1

ⒸJapanese Society for Cancer of the Colon and Rectum 2019
Published 2019 by Kanehara & Co., Ltd.

This English edition is based on the original edition in Japanese:
 "Japanese Classification of Colorectal, Appendiceal, and Anal Carcinoma"(9th edition) edited by Japanese Society for Cancer of the Colon and Rectum, which is published by Kanehara & Co., Ltd.
ⒸJapanese Society for Cancer of the Colon and Rectum 2018
ISBN 978-4-307-20389-0

This work is subject to copyright. All rights are reserved, whether the whole or part of the material is concerned, specifically the rights of translation, reprinting, reuse of illustrations, recitation, broadcasting, reproduction on microfilms or in any other way, and storage in data banks.
Duplication of this publication or parts thereof is only permitted under the provision of the Japanese Copyright Law in its current version, and a copyright fee must always be paid. Violations fall under the prosecution act of the Japanese Copyright Law.
The use of registered names, trademarks, etc., in this publication does not imply, even in the absence of a specific statement, that such names are exempt from the relevant protective laws and regulations and therefore free for general use.
Product Liability: The publisher can give no guarantee for information about drug dosage and application thereof contained in this book. In every individual case the respective user must check its accuracy by consulting other pharmaceutical literature.

Kanehara & Co., Ltd.
31-14, 2-Chome, Yushima, Bunkyo-ku, Tokyo, 113-0034, Japan
http://www.kanehara-shuppan.co.jp/

Printed in Japan

Japanese Society for Cancer of the Colon and Rectum
  Samban-cho KS building, Samban-cho 2, Chiyoda-city, Tokyo, 102-0075, Japan

English Edition Committee, Chairman
  Masafumi Inomata

English Edition Committee Members
  Kenjiro Kotake, Yoichi Ajioka, Kazushige Kawai, Hideki Ueno, Takanori Goi,
  Kentaro Nakajima, Tomonori Akagi

Adviser for the English Edition Commitee
  Hideaki Yano

Japanese Edition Committee, Chairman
  Kenichi Sugihara

Japanese Edition Committee Members
  Yoichi Ajioka, Tsutomu Chiba, Takahiro Fujimori, Hiroharu Isomoto, Shingo Ishiguro,
  Masaaki Ito, Akinori Iwashita, Yukihide Kanemitsu, Tomoyuki Kato, Tomoe Katsumata,
  Yusuke Kinugasa, Susumu Kodaira, Fumio Konishi, Kenjiro Kotake, Yasuo Koyama,
  Shin-ei Kudo, Ryoji Kushima, Masaki Mori, Takeo Mori, Yoshihiro Moriya, Kei Muro,
  Tetsuichiro Muto, Atsushi Ochiai, Kiyotaka Okuno, Masatoshi Ohya, Yutaka Saito,
  Yoshihiro Sakai, Yoshiharu Satake, Yasuhiro Shimada, Kazuo Shirouzu, Tamotsu Sugai,
  Akinori Takagane, Shinji Tanaka, Kazutaka Yamada, Takashi Yao, Masayuki Yasutomi

Japanese Revision Edition Committee, Chairman
  Kenjiro Kotake

Japanese Revision Edition Committee Members
  Yoichi Ajioka, Hideki Ueno, Masazumi Okajima, Atsushi Ochiai, Yukihide Kanemitsu,
  Ryoji Kushima, Keiji Yukita, Hirotoshi Kobayashi, Yutaka Saito, Yasuhiro Shimada, Shinji Tanaka,
  Yojiro Hashiguchi, Kazuo Hase, Tetsuya Hamaguchi, Kotaro Maeda, Takashi Yao,
  Kazutaka Yamada, Toshiaki Watanabe, Masahiko Watanabe

Preface of the Third English Edition

The Japanese Society for Cancer of the Colon and Rectum (JSCCR) is pleased to publish the third English edition of the Japanese Classification of Colorectal, Appendiceal and Anal Carcinoma (JCCRC), which is the translated version of the ninth Japanese edition of the JCCRC published in July 2018. The previous English edition published in January 2009 is the translated version of the seventh Japanese edition of JCCRC.

Our classification and treatment strategies for colorectal cancer, which have been developed based on accumulating clinical and histopathological studies on colorectal cancer in patients treated during a span of 45 years in Japan, differ from those implemented in Western countries in certain regards. Similar to trends observed in industry, economy, society, and culture, among others, medical care is also affected by globalization. The latest edition of the JCCRC is focused on harmonization with the TNM classification. However, several differences still exist, which stem from unique and detailed surgical approaches and histopathological studies, such as those involving main lymph nodes around the feeding arteries, lateral lymph nodes on the pelvic side wall for rectal cancer, and extramural discontinuous cancer spread and tumor budding. We believe that these are important aspects for a more precise evaluation of the spread in colorectal cancer and a more proper estimation of prognosis.

Furthermore, strategies and recommendations for treatment of colorectal cancer, which were included in the JCCRC before 2005, when the first edition of the Japanese guidelines for treatment of colorectal cancer was published, have been moved to the guidelines for the JCCRC because the Japanese guidelines for colorectal cancer have been improved through several editions since 2005.

The number of clinical and histopathological studies on colorectal cancer conducted in Japan and published in English medical journals has been increasing significantly. Most of these studies rely on data collected according to the JCCRC. Publication of the English version of the recently revised JCCRC will contribute immensely toward a better understanding of these articles by non-Japanese readers.

February 2019

Kenichi Sugihara
President,
Japanese Society for Cancer of the Colon and Rectum

Preface of the Second English Edition

Thirty-five years have passed since the Japanese Society for Cancer of the Colon and Rectum (JSCCR) was first established in 1973. During this period, the incidence of colorectal cancer has increased 4.5 fold in Japan. Consequently, Japan has one of the highest incidences of colorectal cancer in the world. The first edition of the General Rules of Japanese Classification of Colorectal Carcinoma (JCCRC) was published in Japanese in 1977 and the latest edition (7th edition) in 2006. Our classification system and treatment strategy of colorectal cancer differ in some respects from those of western countries; particularly, in grouping and grading of regional lymph nodes, grading of lymph node dissection and management of early cancer. Over a period of 35 years, our treatment strategies have undergone substantial development with advances in diagnostic imaging and an accumulation of experience based on analysis of the database of JSCCR, which has been reflected in each new edition.

In the 7th Japanese edition, considerable changes have been made to enhance consistency both with TNM classification and with Japanese classifications of other gastrointestinal cancers. In addition, the part relating to treatment strategies has been excluded from the 7th edition as the JSCCR guidelines for the treatment of colorectal cancer were published in 2005. All histopathologic micrographs of various types of tumors have been renewed and macroscopic and colonoscopic photographs of tumors of each macroscopic type have been updated in an attempt to help share uniform pictures of the classification of tumor appearances.

As more than 10 years have passed since the first English edition was translated from the 5th Japanese edition, we have decided to publish the English version of the latest edition. The current edition of JCCRC is intended to clarify for foreign clinicians and pathologists the underlying principles of the current Japanese classification system and how they are being continuously developed upon to further improve quality of diagnosis and prognosis of colorectal cancer.

January 2009

Kenichi Sugihara
President,
Japanese Society for Cancer of the Colon and Rectum

Preface of the First English Edition

In 1977, the Japanese Society for Cancer of the Colon and Rectum published the first Japanese edition of the General Rules for Clinical and Pathological Studies on Cancer of the Colon, Rectum, and Anus. Goals of the General Rules were to contribute to the continuing investigation and treatments of these cancers by applying common rules of clinical and pathological descriptions. Since the TNM classification by the UICC was not yet established at the time, the General Rules were prepared based on the Dukes classification and other general rules by Japanese societies, such as the Japanese Research Society for Gastric Cancer, the Japanese Society for Breast Cancer, the Japanese Society for Esophageal Diseases, and etc. However, the need for details and accurate descriptions in the General Rules impressed to be a high-level science but a complex practice. We believe that they have been achieving their intended goal and that they are indispensable.

The General Rules have always tried to meet three requirements: 1) to be simple, universally applicable, and useful; 2) to be adequate for statistical studies; and 3) to be internationally acceptable. Furthermore, we thought that the General Rules, which should be theoretical and systematic as a manual, would not be of much benefit unless their concepts became diffused. According to this policy, part of the 3rd edition was translated into English in the Japanese Journal of Surgery (1983), which has been well received and utilized.

The General Rules repeated corrections and revisions cover classifications of clinical and histopathological aspects, including aspects of surgical treatments, endoscopy, radiotherapy, and chemotherapy. In particular, regional lymph nodes have been grouped, according to anatomical distance from the tumor, for the advancement of surgical treatments. This seemingly complex concept is presumed to be useful for understanding tumor invasion and lymph node dissection. In addition, improvement of the curability of distant metastases to the liver and lungs is expected to result from surgical resections. The categories of regional lymph nodes and the curability are also included in the General Rules.

Now, we present the first English edition of the Japanese Classification of Colorectal Carcinoma, with full illustrations and detailed descriptions. This English edition is based on the 5th Japanese edition of the General Rules.

I sincerely hope that this English edition will be widely accepted, and that it will contribute to treatments of colorectal cancer.

October 1997

Masayuki Yasutomi
President,
Japanese Society for Cancer of the Colon and Rectum

Table of Contents

The principles of revision and changes from the previous edition (the 8th Japanese edition). ... *1*

I. Guidelines for classification ... *5*
1 Aims and subjects ... *6*
   1.1 Aims ... *6*
   1.2 Subjects ... *6*
2 General principles of description methods ... *6*
   2.1 Clinical, surgical, and pathological findings ... *6*
   2.2 Findings following preoperative treatment ... *7*
   2.3 Findings of recurrence ... *7*
3 Recording of findings ... *7*
   3.1 Primary tumors ... *7*
      3.1.1 Tumor location ... *7*
      3.1.2 Anatomical divisions of colon and rectum, vermiform appendix, and anal canal ... *7*
      3.1.3 Circumferential divisions of the wall of the rectum and anal canal ... *10*
      3.1.4 Number and size of lesions and proportion of the tumor in relation to the circumference of the bowel ... *10*
      3.1.5 Macroscopic types ... *10*
         3.1.5.1 Main macroscopic types ... *10*
         3.1.5.2 Subtypes of macroscopic type 0 ... *11*
      3.1.6 Depth of tumor invasion (T) ... *12*
   3.2 Metastasis ... *13*
      3.2.1 Lymph node metastasis ... *13*
         3.2.1.1 Lymph node groups and station numbers ... *13*
         3.2.1.2 Lymph node station number ... *13*
         3.2.1.3 Regional lymph nodes ... *14*
         3.2.1.4 Lymph node metastasis (N) ... *17*
      3.2.2 Distant metastasis (M) ... *17*
         3.2.2.1 Liver metastasis (H) ... *18*
         3.2.2.2 Peritoneal metastasis (P) ... *19*
         3.2.2.3 Pulmonary metastasis (PUL) ... *19*
   3.3 Stage grouping ... *20*
      3.3.1 Clinical and pathological classifications for stage grouping ... *20*
      3.3.2 Stage grouping following preoperative treatment ... *22*
   3.4 Multiple colorectal cancers, multiple primary cancers ... *22*
   3.5 Family history and hereditary diseases ... *22*

4 Endoscopic and surgical treatments — 23
4.1 Endoscopic treatment — 23
4.1.1 Endoscopic treatment method — 23
4.2 Surgical treatment — 24
4.2.1 Approach to the lesion — 24
4.2.2 Surgical procedures — 24
4.2.3 Lymph node dissection — 25
4.2.3.1 Extent of lymph node dissection (D) — 25
4.2.3.2 Extent of lateral lymph node dissection (LD) — 26
4.2.4 Anastomosis — 26
4.2.4.1 Types of anastomosis — 26
4.2.4.2 Methods of anastomosis — 27
4.2.5 Combined resection of adjacent organs and structures — 27
4.2.6 Preservation of autonomic nerves (AN) — 27

5 Assessment of cancer involvement at resected margin, residual tumor, and curability — 28
5.1 Cancer involvement at resection margins — 28
5.1.1 Specimens obtained by endoscopic resection — 28
5.1.1.1 Horizontal margin (lateral/mucosal margin) (HM) — 28
5.1.1.2 Vertical margin (deep/intramural margin) (VM) — 28
5.1.2 Specimens obtained by surgical resection — 29
5.1.2.1 Proximal margin (PM) — 29
5.1.2.2 Distal margin (DM) — 29
5.1.2.3 Radial margin (circumferential resection margin) (RM) — 29
5.2 Residual tumor — 29
5.2.1 Residual tumor following endoscopic treatment (ER) — 29
5.2.2 Residual tumor following surgical treatment (R) — 29
5.3 Curability — 30

6 Chemotherapy and radiotherapy — 31
6.1 Chemotherapy documentation — 31
6.2 Radiotherapy documentation — 31
6.2.1 Aims of radiotherapy — 31
6.2.2 Methods of radiotherapy — 31
6.2.3 Radiation field — 31

7 Evaluation of resected specimens — 32
7.1 Macroscopic findings — 32
7.1.1 Tumor location — 32
7.1.2 Macroscopic types — 32
7.1.3 Size — 32
7.1.3.1 Tumor size — 32
7.1.3.2 Size of the intramucosal component of the tumor — 32
7.1.3.3 Size of the ulcerated area — 32

    7.1.4 Proportion of the tumor in relation to the circumference of the bowel *32*
    7.1.5 Distance from the lesion to the resection margin *32*
    7.1.6 Extent and properties of invasion and metastasis *32*
    7.1.7 Depth of tumor invasion *32*
    7.1.8 Lymph node metastasis and location *32*
7.2 Histological findings *32*
    7.2.1 Histological types *32*
        A. Colon and rectum *32*
        B. Vermiform appendix *34*
        C. Anal canal (including the perianal skin) *34*
    7.2.2 Infiltration pattern (INF) *35*
    7.2.3 Lymphovascular invasion *35*
        7.2.3.1 Lymphatic invasion (Ly) *35*
        7.2.3.2 Venous invasion (V) *36*
    7.2.4 Tumor budding (BD) *36*
    7.2.5 Extramural cancer deposits without lymph node structure (EX) *37*
    7.2.6 Perineural invasion (Pn) *37*
7.3 Histological criteria for the assessment of response to chemotherapy/
    rediotherapy *38*
7.4 Histological assessment of biopsy specimens
    (Group classification) *39*
7.5 Measurement of the depth of invasion *39*
    7.5.1 T1 cancer *39*
    7.5.2 Tumor invasion beyond the MP in sites without the serosa *40*

8 Treatment outcome record *40*
8.1 Number of patients *40*
8.2 Multiple colorectal cancers, multiple primary cancers *41*
8.3 Modalities of treatment and adjuvant therapy *41*
8.4 Total number of colorectal cancer cases with treatment, and the
    number and rate of cases by treatment types *41*
    8.4.1 Resection rate *41*
    8.4.2 Endoscopic treatment *41*
    8.4.3 Chemotherapy and radiotherapy *41*
8.5 Number and rate of operative mortality *41*
8.6 Number and rate of hospital mortality following surgery *42*
8.7 Survival analysis *42*
    8.7.1 Survival *42*
    8.7.2 Recurrence/metastasis; site(s) and mode *42*
    8.7.3 Survival analysis method *43*

Supplement: Lymph node groups and station number *44*
Supplementary Reference of Macroscopic Types *47*

Supplement: Measurement of submucosal invasion distance ········· 56

II. Assessment of response to chemotherapy and radiotherapy
.... 57
1 Assessment of response ··· 58
2 Definition of efficacy endpoints ·· 58
    2.1 Response rate ··· 58
    2.2 Overall survival (OS), progression-free survival (PFS), relapse-free survival (RFS), disease-free survival (DFS), time to treatment failure (TTF) ··· 58
3 Documentation of adverse events ··· 59

III. Explanation of pathological items [Supplement: Histology Atlas] ··· 61
1 Histological types ··· 62
    A. Colon and rectum ·· 62
    B. Vermiform appendix ·· 71
    C. Anal canal (including the perianal skin) ··· 72
2 Histological assessment of biopsy specimens (Group classification) ········· 74
3 Handling of resected specimens ·· 76
    3.1 Handling of biopsy materials ·· 76
    3.2 Macroscopic examination and handling of surgically resected specimens ··· 76
    3.3 Handling of endoscopically resected specimens ································· 79
Supplementary histology atlas ·· 81

Supplements ·· 103
    Supplement 1 TNM Classification of malignant tumours ····················· 104
        Supplement-1-1 Carcinoma of the colon and rectum ······················· 104
        Supplement 1-2 Carcinoma of the appendix ···································· 108
        Supplement 1-3 Carcinoma of the anal canal ·································· 110
        Supplement 1-4 Well-differentiated neuroendocrine tumours (G1 and G2) of the colon and rectum, and the appendix ································ 112
    Supplement 2 Summary of findings ··· 114
    Supplement 3 Checklist for pathological report ·································· 116
    Supplement 4 List of abbreviations ··· 118

Index ··· 120

The principles of revision and changes from the previous edition (the 8th Japanese edition).

Through defining detailed rules for evaluating and documenting clinical and pathological findings and handling specimens of colorectal cancer, the Japanese Classification of Colorectal, Appendiceal, and Anal Carcinoma (JCCRC), published by Japanese Society for Cancer of the Colon and Rectum (JSCCR), has contributed to the standardization and improvement of the diagnosis and treatment of colorectal cancer in Japan. Furthermore, the JSCCR guidelines for colorectal cancer treatment, which has been revised several times since its first edition issued in 2005, describe treatment algorithms that conform to the Japanese classification; therefore, its importance is continuing to increase. Under these circumstances, the revisions have to serve to maintain the role of the classification to further improve treatment outcomes for colorectal cancer in Japan, which are already one of the best in the world. At the same time, there is a focus on harmonizing with the eighth edition of the TNM classification (2017) and classification of cancers in other organs in Japan.

Stage grouping of colorectal cancer was compromised with that of the TNM classification. However, some differences are caused by the classification of lymph node metastasis. Expertise built up over several years emphasize on the importance of the main and lateral lymph nodes (N3) in Japan. Further, the definition of "extramural discontinuous cancer spread (EX)" differs from that of "tumor deposits" in the TNM classifications. Meanwhile, because of the low prevalence of appendiceal and anal cancers arising from the anoderm in Japan, the current edition incorporates the TNM classification in these clinical entities.

Changes between the previous (the 8th Japanese edition) and current editions are described below:

Ⅰ. Guidelines for classification
2 General principles of description methods

For "Stage" of appendiceal and anal cancers, Roman numerals and uppercase alphabets are used (*e.g.*, Stage ⅢA).

For "Stage" of colorectal cancer, Roman numerals and lowercase alphabets are used (*e.g.*, Stage Ⅲa) (Page 6).

3 Recording of findings
3.1.6 Depth of tumor invasion (T)

T category of rectal-type anal cancers has been redefined (Page 12).

The definition of pT4a has been changed (Page 12).

3.2.1.4 Lymph node metastasis (N)
N1 is now divided into N1a and N1b, and N2 is divided into N2a and N2b (Page 17).

3.2.2 Distant metastasis (M)
Distant metastasis (M1) is reclassified as M1a–M1c in accordance with the TNM classification (Eighth edition). M1c is now divided into M1c1 (metastasis to the peritoneum only) and M1c2 (metastasis to the peritoneum with other organs) (Page 17).

3.2.2.2 Peritoneal metastasis (P)
Ovarian metastasis is categorized as distant metastasis and recorded using the symbol "OVA." For example, a single ovarian metastasis would be recorded as M1a (OVA) (Page 19).

3.3.1 Clinical and pathological classification for stage grouping
Stage grouping of colorectal cancer has been revised. Stage II is now subdivided into stages IIa–IIc, Stage III into stages IIIa–IIIc, and Stage IV into stages IVa–IVc (Page 20).

3.4 Multiple colorectal cancers, multiple primary cancers
Simultaneous occurrences of cancers are now defined as "diagnosis within a period of less than 2 months," whereas metachronous occurrences are now defined as "diagnosis within a period of 2 months or more" (Page 22).

4.1.1 Endoscopic treatment method
Cold forceps polypectomy, cold snare polypectomy, precutting endoscopic mucosal resection (EMR), and hybrid endoscopic submucosal dissection (ESD) have been included in the notes (Page 23).

4.2.2 Surgical procedures
Definitions of ultra-low anterior and intersphincteric resections and standard surgical procedures for familial adenomatous polyposis are included in the notes (Page 24).

4.2.3 Lymph node dissection
In lower rectal cancers as well as in those cancers with infiltration reaching to the lower rectum, dissection of lymph nodes along the major named vessels and bowel axis (D) should be

recorded separately from the lateral node dissections (LDs).
Extent of LD has been newly defined (LDX–LD3) (Page 25, 26).

5.2.1 Residual tumor following endoscopic treatment (ER)
ER1 is now classified into ER1a (HM1 and VM0) and ER1b (HM0, VM1, or HM1 VM1) (Page 29).

7.2.1 Histological types
Carcinoid tumors and endocrine cell carcinomas are now separated from endocrine tumors and individually subclassified within malignant epithelial tumors (Page 32).

7.2.2 Infiltration pattern (INF)
Judgment methods have been revised from "using the naked eye" to "loupe images or low magnification" (Page 35).

7.2.3 Lymphovascular invasion
The abbreviation for lymphatic invasion has been changed from "ly" to "Ly" and that for venous invasion has been changed from "v" to "V." The extent of invasion is now expressed using Ly1a–Ly1c and V1a–V1c. Further, V2 is now defined as macroscopic venous invasion (Page 35).

7.2.4 Tumor budding (BD)
Tumor budding is now abbreviated as "BD" (Page 36).

7.2.6 Perineural invasion (Pn)
The abbreviation for perineural invasion has been revised from "PN" to "Pn" (Page 37).

7.5 Measurement of the depth of invasion
7.5.1 T1 cancer
"Supplementary figures: Measurement method of the depth of invasion of T1 cancer" has been newly added (Page 39).

Table 4 Supplement: Lymph node groups and station number
The "external sacral lymph nodes (260)", "median sacral lymph nodes (270)", and "aortic bifurcation lymph nodes (280)" have been revised from "other lymph nodes" to "lateral lymph nodes." The "inguinal lymph nodes" (292) has been revised from "other lymph nodes" to "lower lymph nodes" (Page 44).

II. Assessment of response to chemotherapy and radiotherapy

Descriptions regarding Response Evaluation Criteria in Solid Tumors (RECIST) have been greatly reduced (Page 58).

III. Explanation of pathological items [Supplement: Histology Atlas]

The section of handling of resected specimens has been revised (Pages 76 to 80).
The supplementary histology atlas has been updated (Pages 81 to 101).

Supplement 1. TNM classifications

The comparison table between the TNM and Japanese classifications for colorectal cancer has been updated (Page 106).
TNM classifications for appendiceal and anal cancers are now listed (Page 108, 110).
TNM classifications for colorectal and appendiceal carcinoids have been updated (Page 112, 113).

Supplement 2. Summary of findings

The summary of findings is now updated (Page 114).

Supplement 3. Checklist for pathological report

The checklist has been newly added (Page 116).

Supplement 4 List of abbreviations

The list of abbreviations is now updated (Page 118).

[Deleted Items]

Curability of endoscopic treatments (Cur E)
Histological findings: Interstitial volume (medullary, intermediate, and scirrhous types), endocrine cell tumors.
Pathological atlas: Histological assessment of biopsied specimen (Group classifications).

This revised edition of classification was drafted by the Japanese Revision Edition Committee of the JSCCR and determined on the basis of agreements formed by the Japanese Edition Committee of the JSCCR.
This revised edition will be applicable to cases treated from 2019 onward in the JSCCR colorectal cancer registry.

I. Guidelines for classification

1 Aims and subjects

1.1 Aims
This classification presents anatomical extent of colorectal cancer as a means to broadly share clinicopathological information on colorectal cancer and serves as the basis to improve treatment outcomes for colorectal cancer in Japan.

1.2 Subjects
This classification applies to primary carcinomas of the colon and rectum and does not apply to recurrence or metastasis. It is recommended that findings for primary colorectal tumors other than carcinomas should be recorded according to this classification. The large intestine comprises the colon (cecum, ascending colon, transverse colon, descending colon, and sigmoid colon) and rectum (rectosigmoid junction, upper rectum, and lower rectum). The current edition also pertains to the appendix and anal canal; tumors occurring in these regions are separately tallied from those occurring in the colorectum.

2 General principles of description methods

Findings are recorded using uppercase letters for the extent of primary tumor (T), lymph node metastasis (N), and distant metastasis (M). The degree of each finding is recorded in Arabic numerals following the designated letter. If the degree of findings needs to be subclassified, then it is recorded using lowercase letters placed after the Arabic numeral (*e.g.*, T4a). "X" denotes the absence or uncertainty of assigning a given category (*e.g.*, NX). Staging is recorded using Roman numerals, and subclassifications are recorded using lowercase letters (*e.g.*, Stage IIIa). Staging for appendiceal and anal cancers originating from the squamous epithelium, anal glands, and anal gland ducts is recorded using Roman numerals and subdivision using uppercase alphabets (*e.g.*, Stage IIIA).

2.1 Clinical, surgical, and pathological findings
Categories of findings, i.e., clinical, surgical, and pathological, are identified by placing the lowercase letters "c," "s," and "p," respectively, in front of the designated finding.
Clinical findings: physical findings, diagnostic imaging findings, and biopsy/cytology as a preoperative diagnosis
Surgical findings: surgical and diagnostic imaging findings during surgery.
Pathological findings: pathological findings of specimens obtained by endoscopic and/or surgical treatments, including intraoperative and rapid intraoperative cytology.

2.2 Findings following preoperative treatment

Findings following preoperative treatment are identified by the prefix "y."
Clinical findings following preoperative treatment are identified by "yc," and pathological findings following preoperative treatment are identified by "yp."

2.3 Findings of recurrence

Findings of recurrence are identified by the prefix "r."
Examples: Clinical findings rT0N0M1a (H); pathological findings rT0N0pM1a (H).

3 Recording of findings

3.1 Primary tumors

3.1.1 Tumor location

The location of cancer is recorded in accordance with the anatomical division of the large intestine. For rectal and anal cancers, the circumferential division of the intestinal wall is recorded.

3.1.2 Anatomical divisions of colon and rectum, vermiform appendix, and anal canal (Page 9, Fig. 1)

Colon

  C: Cecum

   The pouch-like region extending caudal to the upper lip of the ileocecal valve. The boundary with the ascending colon is at the height of the upper lip of the ileocecal valve.

  A: Ascending colon

   The segment that extends from the cecum to the right colic flexure

  T: Transverse colon

   The segment that extends between the left and right colic flexures

  D: Descending colon

   The segment fixed to the retroperitoneum extending from the left colic flexure to the root of the sigmoid colon (approximately at the height of the iliac crest)

  S: Sigmoid colon

   The segment extending from the descending colon to the height of the sacral promontory.

Rectum

  RS: Rectosigmoid

   The segment from the height of the sacral promontory to the inferior border of the second sacral vertebra

Ra: Upper rectum

The segment from the height of the inferior border of the second sacral vertebra to the peritoneal reflection

Rb: Lower rectum

The segment from the peritoneal reflection to the superior border of the puborectal sling.

Note 1: The tubular portion corresponding to the ileocecal valve (transitional portion from the ileum to the cecum) is included in the cecum.

Note 2: It is not consistent worldwide whether the intestinal tract from the sacral promontory to the inferior border of the second sacral vertebra is included in either the colon or the rectum; however, in this classification, it is called RS and treated as the rectum.

Note 3: If more than one division is involved, then each division involved is recorded in the order of degree of involvement, starting with the division in which the bulk of the tumor is located.

e.g.: RS-Ra

Note 4: For rectal cancer, the distance between the lower edge of the tumor and the anal verge or dentate line is recorded. The anal verge is the connection between the anoderm and hair-bearing skin.

V: Vermiform appendix

Note: The TNM classification scheme described on Page 108 is used for the classification of tumors originating in the appendix.

P: Anal canal

The "anal canal" can be described either as the surgical or anatomical anal canal. The surgical anal canal corresponds to the tubular structure extending from the superior border of the puborectal sling to the anal verge, whereas the anatomical anal canal corresponds to the tubular structure covered by the anoderm from the dentate line to the anal verge. The current JCCRC refers to the surgical anal canal (Fig. 2).

Note: Types of cancer that develop in the anal canal include those that originate from the mucosa of the rectal part of the anal canal (rectal type adenocarcinoma) and those that originate from the squamous epithelium of the anal canal, the anal gland, or a duct of it (squamous cell carcinoma, anal gland carcinoma, carcinoma associated with fistula). The former type anal canal cancer was described considering it as colorectal cancer, and for the description of the latter type, the TNM classifications shown on page 110 was used.

[Extra]

E: Perianal skin

Perianal skin defined as hair-bearing skin within 5 cm of the anal verge (excluding the external genitalia).

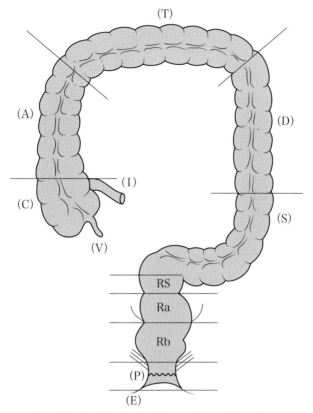

Fig. 1 Anatomical divisions of large intestine

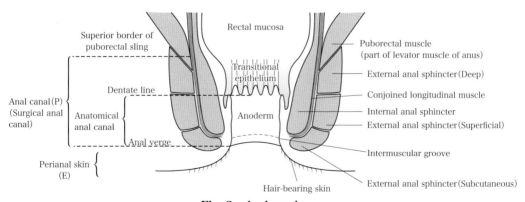

Fig. 2 Anal canal

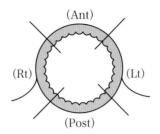

Fig. 3 Proctorectal wall divisions

3.1.3 Circumferential divisions of the wall of the rectum and anal canal (Fig. 3)

The circumference of the wall of the rectum and anal canal is anatomically divided into quadrants as anterior wall (Ant), posterior wall (Post), left wall (Lt), and right wall (Rt). Tumors located in the entire circumference are recorded as "Circ."

> *Note*: If the tumor occupies more than one quadrant, then the primary quadrant is recorded first, *e.g.*, Ant-Lt

3.1.4 Number and size of lesions and proportion of the tumor in relation to the circumference of the bowel

The maximum dimension of the primary tumor, associated maximum perpendicular dimension, and proportion of the tumor in relation to the circumference of the bowel (the percentage of the maximum transverse diameter of the tumor occupying the circumference of the bowel) are recorded. All modalities used for these measurements (such as barium enema, colonoscopy, CT, MRI, ultrasonography, and palpation) are recorded. If the number and size cannot be assessed, then it is recorded as "unknown."

In multiple tumors, the location, size, proportion in relation to the bowel circumference, macroscopic type, and extent of primary tumor are recorded for each tumor. The primary lesion is defined as the lesion with the deepest wall invasion or that with the largest diameter when the depths of wall invasion are the same.

3.1.5 Macroscopic types (Pages 47–52, Fig. 10–15)

3.1.5.1 Main macroscopic types

Type 0: Superficial type
Type 1: Polypoid type
Type 2: Ulcerated type with clear margin
Type 3: Ulcerated type with infiltration
Type 4: Diffusely infiltrating type

Type 5: Unclassified type

3.1.5.2 Subtypes of macroscopic type 0
Type 0-I : Protruded type
 0-Ip: Pedunculated type
 0-Isp: Subpedunculated type
 0-Is: Sessile type
Type 0-II : Superficial type
 0-IIa: Elevated type
 0-IIb: Flat type
 0-IIc: Depressed type

Note 1: Lesions presumed to be Tis and T1 cancers are classified as superficial type (type 0).
Note 2: Endoscopic findings are given priority when diagnosing superficial type lesions. The shape of the lesion is perceived as a whole image, irrespective of histogenesis and neoplastic or non-neoplastic difference.
Note 3: It is difficult to distinguish between adenomas and cancers based on macroscopic findings; therefore, the subclassification of superficial type is also used for the macroscopic classification of adenomatous lesions.
Note 4: If the tumor presents 2 different elements of superficial type, then the type occupying the largest area is recorded first, followed by "+," *e.g.*, 0-IIc + IIa.
Note 5: Laterally spreading tumors (LSTs) describes tumors that have grown (laterally) to more than 10 mm in diameter on the surface and are not included in the macroscopic classification. LSTs are divided according to morphology into granular (G) (homogenous and nodular mixed types) and non-granular (NG) types (flat elevated and pseudodepressed types) (Pages 53–55, Figs. 16 and 17).
Note 6: The macroscopic type must remain unchanged according to the results of the histopathological examination, *e.g.*, superficial lesions remain type 0 even for histologically advanced cancers.
Note 7: Among anal tumors, those that originate from the anal glands or ducts of the anal canal wall and predominantly occupy the muscular layer or beyond are defined as "extra-canal type," whereas those classified as either type 0, 1, 2, 3, 4, or 5 are defined as "intra-canal type."
Note 8: In the event of chemotherapy or radiotherapy, macroscopic types before and after treatment are recorded.

3.1.6 Depth of tumor invasion (T)

TX: Primary tumor cannot be assessed

T0: No evidence of primary tumor

Tis: Tumor is confined to the mucosa (M) and does not invade the submucosa (SM)

T1: Tumor is confined to the SM and does not invade the muscularis propria (MP)

    T1a: Tumor is confined to the SM, and invasion is within 1000 μm

    T1b: Tumor is confined to the SM, and invasion is 1000 μm or more, but it does not extend to the MP (Page 39, 7.5.1 Measurement of the depth of invasion)

T2: Tumor invasion to, but not beyond, the MP

T3: Tumor invades beyond the MP. In sites with serosa, the tumor grows into the subserosa (SS). In sites with no serosa, the tumor grows into the adventitia (A) (Page 40, 7.5.2 Measurement of the depth of invasion)

T4: Tumor invades or perforates the serosa (SE) or directly invades other organs or structures (SI/AI)

    T4a: Tumor invades or perforates the serosa (SE)

    T4b: Tumor directly invades adjacent organs or structures (SI/AI)

Note 1: The extent of invasion of the primary tumor is recorded according to the T classification. Invasion into each layer of the bowel wall and into adjacent organs is denoted using the letters M, SM, MP, SS, A, and SI/AI. SI indicates invasion through the serosa into adjacent organs in sites with the serosa, and AI indicates invasion into adjacent organs in sites with no serosa.

Note 2: In the portion without the serosa, the adventitia (A) describes the pericolic/perirectal tissues equivalent to the SS of the portion with the serosa.

Note 3: The prefixes "c" (clinical findings) and "p" (pathological findings) are only used for the T classification and not for M–SI/AI (pathologically diagnosed mucosal cancer is recorded as pTis, and not pM).

Note 4: Tis conventionally refers to carcinoma in situ without invasion into the lamina propria; however, in colorectal cancer, Tis refers to cancer not extending beyond the lamina propria (i.e., intramucosal carcinoma) regardless of invasion.

Note 5: Regardless of the existence of metastasis, Tis and T1 are designated as "early cancers," and cancers that have grown into the MP or beyond are designated as "advanced cancers." The globally used terms "early stage colorectal cancer" and "advanced colorectal cancer" refer to stages I–III colorectal cancers and unresectable colorectal cancers, respectively, which define stages differently from T classification.

Note 6: For pT4b, the organ invaded is also noted, *e.g.*, pT4b (prostate).

Note 7: The extent of histopathological depth is evaluated using the deepest area of cancer invasion. In case the deepest area is vascular/nerve invasion, it should be noted.

    Example 1: If the cancer invasion is of the proper muscle layer and venous invasion is observed in the SS, then the correct designation is pT3(V)-MP (Page 81, Fig. 22).

Example 2: If the cancer invasion is of the SM, the submucosal invasion distance is 1500 μm, and lymphatic vessel invasion is observed in the SS, then the correct designation is pT3(Ly)-SM: 1500 μm.

Note 8: The definition of the extent of primary tumors has been determined to be consistent with that of other digestive system tumors.

Note 9: TNM classifications take no account of vascular invasion into T classification; consequently, the extent of primary tumor in the TNM classification and the current JCCRC may not agree in a low number of cases. A table comparing the current JCCRC with TNM classifications is provided on pages 106 and 107.

Note 10: The extent of primary tumor of rectal-type anal adenocarcinomas is defined as follows:

TX: Primary tumor cannot be assessed

T0: No evidence of primary tumor

Tis: Tumor is confined to the mucosa (M) and does not extend to the submucosa (SM)

T1: Tumor is confined to SM and does not extend to the internal sphincter

    T1a: Tumor is confined to SM, and the distance of submucosal invasion is less than 1000 μm

    T1b: Tumor is confined to SM, and the distance of submucosal invasion is 1000 μm or greater

T2: Tumor extends to the internal anal sphincter but not to the conjoined longitudinal muscle

T3: Tumor has invaded beyond the conjoined longitudinal muscle

T4: Tumor has invaded the levator ani muscles or adjacent organs or structures

3.2 Metastasis
3.2.1 Lymph node metastasis
3.2.1.1 Lymph node groups and station numbers

Lymph node groups are classified and numbered according to their anatomical relationship to the superior mesenteric, inferior mesenteric, and iliac arteries as shown on pages 44 and 46, Table 4, and Figure 9.

3.2.1.2 Lymph node station number

Lymph node station of the large intestine is indicated with 3-digit numbers in the 200's.
For lymph nodes of the superior and inferior mesenteric arteries, the first digit represents the group, with pericolic lymph nodes denoted by "1," intermediate lymph nodes by "2," and main lymph nodes by "3." The second digit represents the main artery, with the ileocolic

artery denoted by "0," right colic artery by "1," middle colic artery by "2," left colic artery by "3," sigmoid artery by "4," and inferior mesenteric artery along with the superior rectal artery by "5."

Internal iliac lymph nodes are denoted by "P" for central nodes and "D" for peripheral nodes. Internal iliac lymph nodes are identified by "3" for the first digit indicating the group, with "rt" for the right side and "lt" for the left side. As an exception to this convention, lymph nodes in contact with the anterior surface of the sacrum are identified by "0," and inguinal lymph nodes classified as intermediate lymph nodes in anal cancer are identified by "2."

For consistency with the classification of gastric carcinoma, superior mesenteric, para-aortic, sub-pyloric, omental, and splenic hilar lymph nodes are numbered 214, 216, 206, 204, and 210, respectively.

3.2.1.3 Regional lymph nodes

Lymph nodes are divided into regional lymph nodes and others. The presence or absence of regional lymph node metastasis and the degree of metastasis are recorded using the classification N0–N3.

Regional lymph nodes are classified into 3 groups as pericolic, intermediate, and main lymph nodes. In addition, lateral lymph nodes are included in the lower rectum (Fig. 4).

The specific range of regional lymph nodes is individually defined according to the anatomical relationship between the location of the tumor and its main feeding artery/arteries (Fig. 5).

The main arteries of the colon are the ileocolic, right colic, middle colic (right and left branches), left colic, and sigmoid arteries. The range of pericolic lymph nodes in the colon can be classified into the following 4 types on the basis of the positional relationship with the tumor and feeding artery (Fig. 5).

- a: When the feeding artery is directly below the tumor, the area extends 10 cm in both oral and anal directions from the tumor margin.
- b: When there is one feeding artery within 10 cm from the tumor margin, the area extends up to 5 cm beyond the arterial inflow site and the opposite side extends up to 10 cm from the tumor margin.
- c: When there are 2 dominant arteries within 10 cm from the tumor margin, the area extends up to 5 cm beyond the arterial inflow site in both oral and anal sides.
- d: When there are no feeding arteries within 10 cm from the tumor margin, the area extends up to 5 cm beyond the artery closest to the tumor margin and the opposite side extends up to 10 cm from the tumor margin.

In the rectum, the main lymph node is number 253, and the intermediate lymph node is num-

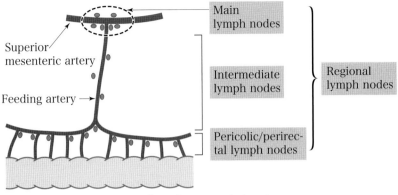
a. Superior mesenteric artery

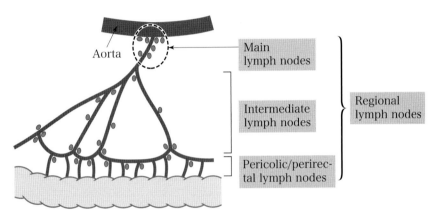
b. Inferior mesenteric artery

Fig. 4 Basic principles of lymph node grouping

ber 252. Pericolic lymph nodes include those between the lowest sigmoid artery inflow point and 3 cm (RS and Ra) or 2 cm (Rb) distal to the tumor margin. However, if the distance from the tumor margin to the lowest sigmoid artery inflow point is less than 10 cm, then pericolic lymph nodes include those in the area up to 10 cm (Fig. 6).

16   I. Guidelines for classification

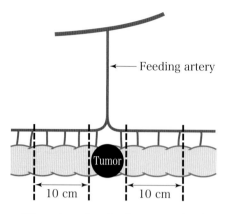

a. When there is a feeding artery in close proximity to the tumor

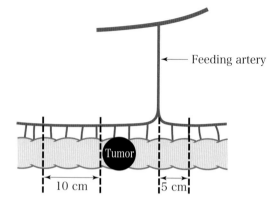

b. When there is only one feeding artery within 10 cm from the tumor margin

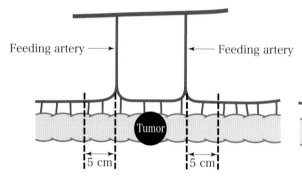

c. When there are 2 dominant arteries within 10 cm from the tumor margin

d. When there are no feeding arteries within 10 cm from the tumor margin, the artery closest to the tumor is regarded as its feeding artery

Fig. 5   Pericolic lymph nodes

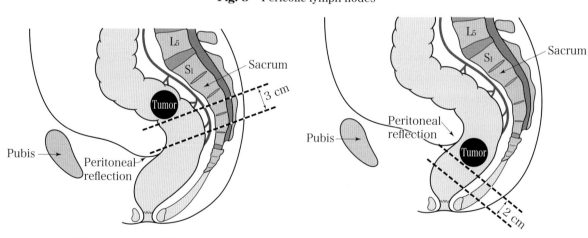

a. When the tumor is located above the peritoneal reflection

b. When the distal edge of the tumor is located below the level of the peritoneal reflection

Fig. 6   Perirectal lymph nodes

3.2.1.4 Lymph node metastasis (N)

NX: Lymph node metastasis cannot be assessed

N0: No evidence of lymph node metastasis

N1: Metastasis in 1–3 pericolic/perirectal or intermediate lymph nodes

   N1a: Metastasis in 1 lymph node

   N1b: Metastasis in 2–3 lymph nodes

N2: Metastasis in 4 or more pericolic/perirectal or intermediate lymph nodes

   N2a: Metastasis in 4–6 lymph nodes

   N2b: Metastasis in 7 or more lymph nodes

N3: Metastasis in the main lymph node(s). In the lower rectal cancer, metastasis in the main and/or lateral lymph node(s)

Note 1: Lymph node metastasis beyond the regional lymph nodes is classified as distant metastasis (M1).

Note 2: Of extramural cancer deposits without lymph node structure (EX), tumor deposits other than vascular/perineural invasion (tumor nodule: ND) are classified as metastatic lymph nodes (Page 37, 7.2.5).

Note 3: The number of dissected and metastatic lymph nodes is described according to the lymph node metastasis ratio (number of metastatic lymph nodes/number of dissected lymph nodes) for each station of the lymph node. The tumor of ND is integrated into that of dissected lymph nodes and the number of ND is discribed.

   Example: If in the 251 area, 3 positive lymph nodes, 2 ND, 1 ND(Pn+), and 5 negative lymph nodes are present, then the designation is #251: 6/11 [ND 2, ND(Pn+) 1].
(Page 37, 7.2.5, *Note 3*)

3.2.2 Distant metastasis (M)

M0: No distant metastasis

M1: Distant metastasis

   M1a: Distant metastasis confined to one organ. Peritoneal metastasis not present

   M1b: Distant metastasis in more than one organ. Peritoneal metastasis not present

M1c: Presence of peritoneal metastasis

   M1c1: Metastasis to the peritoneum only

   M1c2: Metastasis to the peritoneum with other distant metastasis

Note 1: All metastases (lymphogenous, hematogenous, and peritoneal), except for metastasis to the regional lymph nodes, are classified as M1.

Note 2: Ovarian metastasis is now classified as distant metastasis (M1).

Note 3: In the event of hepatic, pulmonary, and peritoneal metastases, the extent of metastasis noted in 3.2.2.1–3.2.2.3 is recorded.

Note 4: In the event of distant metastasis (M1), the site of metastasis is recorded in parentheses. When recording the site of metastasis, the following abbreviations can be used:
Liver: H, Peritoneum: P, Lung: PUL, Bone: OSS, Brain: BRA, Bone marrow: MAR, Adrenal glands: ADR, Skin: SKI, Pleura: PLE, Extraregional lymph nodes: LYM, Ovaries: OVA, Other: OTH
Example M1a (H1), M1a (ADR), M1b (PUL1, H3).

Note 5: With regard to the pathological findings of distant metastasis (pM), "pM0" indicates the absence of distant metastasis confirmed by autopsy and "pM1" indicates histologically confirmed distant metastasis. Accordingly, the diagnosis of distant metastasis based on clinical findings, intraoperative palpation, and/or image findings without histological confirmation are recorded as "cM0" and "cM1." When the pathological findings of distant metastasis are unclear, "pMX" is not used.

3.2.2.1 Liver metastasis (H)

HX: Liver metastasis cannot be assessed

H0: No liver metastasis

H1: 1–4 metastatic tumors, all of which are 5 cm or less in maximum diameter

H2: Other than H1 or H3

H3: Five or more metastatic tumors at least one of which is more than 5 cm in maximum diameter

The prognostic grouping (Grade classification) of patients with liver metastasis is recorded as follows (Table 1):

Grade A: H1 N0/N1

Grade B: H1 N2 or H2 N0/N1

Grade C: Other than the above

Table 1 Grade of patients with liver metastasis

N and M of the primary tumor	H1	H2	H3
N0	A	B	C
N1	A	B	C
N2	B	C	C
N3	C	C	C
M1	C	C	C

Note 1: "N" refers to the grade of lymph node metastasis of the primary tumor.
Note 2: "H" and "Grade" are recorded together, *e.g.*, H1 (Grade A).
Note 3: When nodal status of the primary tumor cannot be assessed, the grade is not determined.

Note 4: Lymph node metastasis to the hepatic hilum is denoted by H-N; if there is no metastasis, then it is recorded as H-N0, and if there is metastasis, then it is recorded as H-N1.

3.2.2.2 Peritoneal metastasis (P)

PX: Peritoneal metastasis cannot be assessed

P0: No peritoneal metastasis

P1: Metastasis localized to adjacent peritoneum

P2: Limited metastasis to distant peritoneum

P3: Diffuse metastasis to distant peritoneum

Note 1: When ascites is present, cytological examination is recommended.

Note 2: Negative results of cytological examination are represented as Cy0 and positive results as Cy1. Cytological examination of ascites is Ⅰ: negative, Ⅲ: false-positive, and Ⅴ: positive, with only positive (Ⅴ) results defined as Cy1.

Note 3: The impact on the prognosis of Cy1 is currently unclear; therefore, Cy1 is not included as a factor to determine staging.

Note 4: The clinical significance of cytological examination of peritoneal lavage fluid has yet to be determined. If the examination is proved to be positive, then the result is recorded as such, but not as Cy1.

3.2.2.3 Pulmonary metastasis (PUL)

PULX: Pulmonary metastasis cannot be assessed

PUL0: No pulmonary metastasis

PUL1: 1 or 2 pulmonary metastases or 3 metastases or more on one side

PUL2: 3 or more pulmonary metastases bilaterally or carcinomatous lymphangitis, carcinomatous pleuritis, and lymph node metastasis in the pulmonary hilum and/or mediastinum

Prognostic grouping (Grade classification) of patients with pulmonary metastasis is recorded as follows (Table 2).

The grade of patients with pulmonary metastasis is determined according to the extent of lymph node metastasis of the primary tumor, distant metastasis, pulmonary metastasis, and disease-free interval (DFI).

Grade A: One pulmonary metastasis, DFI$\geq$2 years, and N0/N1; one pulmonary metastasis, DFI$<$2 years, and N0; 2 pulmonary metastases or 3 or more pulmonary metastases on one side and N0.

Grade B: One pulmonary metastasis, DFI≥2 years, and N2/N3 or M1 (H); one pulmonary metastasis and DFI<2 years; 2 pulmonary metastases or 3 or more pulmonary metastases on one side and N1/N2.

Grade C: Other than the above

DFI is the period from the day of surgery of the primary tumor till the day when pulmonary metastasis is confirmed. For synchronous pulmonary metastasis, DFI is recorded as "0."

Table 2   Grade classification for patients with pulmonary metastasis

N and M of the primary tumor	PUL1		PUL2
	One pulmonary metastasis and DFI≥2 years	Other than on the left	
N0	A		
N1			
N2		B	
N3, M1 (H)			
M1 (except H)			C

Note 1: N is the extent of lymph node metastasis of the primary tumor.
Note 2: PUL and grade are recorded side by side, *e.g.*, PUL1 (Grade A).
Note 3: When nodal status of the primary tumor cannot be assessed, the grade is not determined.
Note 4: Status of lymph node metastasis of the pulmonary hilum and mediastinum is described using PUL-N; negative node is recorded as PUL-N0, and positive node (s) is recorded as PUL-N1.

3.3 Stage grouping (Table 3)

3.3.1 Clinical and pathological classifications for stage grouping

Stage is divided into clinical and pathological classifications, which are denoted by the letters "c" and "p" placed before each respective staging (cStage and pStage).

cStage is based on pretreatment clinical findings and not on surgical findings.

pStage is based on pathological findings. However, clinical findings and/or surgical findings can be used to determine distant metastasis (M) (Page 17).

e.g., Resection of colon cancer without distant metastasis: pT3pN1M0, pStage IIIb

Resection of the primary tumor only in rectal cancer with pulmonary metastasis: pT3pN2M1 (PUL2), pStage IV

Stage 0	Tis	N0	M0
Stage I	T1, T2	N0	M0
Stage II	T3, T4	N0	M0
Stage IIa	T3	N0	M0
Stage IIb	T4a	N0	M0
Stage IIc	T4b	N0	M0
Stage III	Any T	N1, N2, N3	M0
Stage IIIa	T1, T2	N1	M0
	T1	N2a	M0
Stage IIIb	T1, T2	N2b, N3	M0
	T2, T3	N2a	M0
	T3, T4a	N1	M0
Stage IIIc	T3, T4a	N2b, N3	M0
	T4a	N2a	M0
	T4b	N1, N2, N3	M0
Stage IV	Any T	Any N	M1
Stage IVa	Any T	Any N	M1a
Stage IVb	Any T	Any N	M1b
Stage IVc	Any T	Any N	M1c

Table 3 Stage grouping of colorectal cancer

M category		M0				M1		
						M1a	M1b	M1c
N category		N0	N1 (N1a/N1b)	N2a	N2b, N3	Any N		
T	Tis	0						
	T1a・T1b	I	IIIa			IVa	IVb	IVc
	T2			IIIb				
	T3	IIa						
	T4a	IIb			IIIc			
	T4b	IIc						

Stage grouping is possible in the following, even with TX and/or NX.
    TisNXM0　Stage 0
    TXNXM1　Stage IV

3.3.2 Stage grouping following preoperative treatment

Staging following preoperative treatment is designated by the prefix "y" placed before the Roman numeral. The clinical classification following preoperative treatment is designated by "yc," and the pathological classification following preoperative treatment is designated by "yp,"

   e.g., ypT1N1M0 ypStage IIIa.

3.4 Multiple colorectal cancers, multiple primary cancers*

In case of multiple colorectal cancers, the number of lesions is recorded.
In case of multiple primary cancers, the organs involved are recorded.

   Note 1: Presence of Tis cancer is specified in multiple colorectal cancer.
   Note 2: Whether cancers are synchronous or metachronous is recorded.

3.5 Family history and hereditary diseases

For all cancer prevalence in first-degree relatives (parents, children, or siblings) of the patient, the disease name, relationship, sex, and age at diagnosis are recorded. In the event that cancer is found in a first-degree relative of the patient, the disease name, relationship, sex, and age at diagnosis of that individual's first-degree relative are also recorded.

Cases of familial adenomatous polyposis or Lynch syndrome (hereditary non-polyposis colorectal cancer) should be noted**

Reference in footnote: Stage grouping of the TNM classification (Page 104).

M category		M0				M1		
						M1a	M1b	M1c
N category		N0	N1 (N1a/N1b/N1c)	N2a	N2b	Any N		
T category	Tis	0						
	T1	I	IIIA			IVA	IVB	IVC
	T2			IIIB				
	T3	IIA						
	T4a	IIB		IIIC				
	T4b	IIC						

Source: TNM Classification of Malignant Tumours. Eighth Edition, 2017, Wiley-Blackwell, Chichester UK

4 Endoscopic and surgical treatments

4.1 Endoscopic treatment
4.1.1 Endoscopic treatment method
Snare polypectomy
Endoscopic mucosal resection (EMR)
Endoscopic submucosal dissection (ESD)

> *Note 1*: Any other therapeutic procedure, if performed, is recorded.
> *Note 2*: Whether the resection has been performed en bloc or by piecemeal is recorded.
> *Note 3*: Resections that do not utilize high-frequency currents include cold forceps polypectomy and cold snare polypectomy.

---

*Multiple colorectal cancer is defined as the development of two or more primary tumors in the large intestine. Multiple primary cancer is defined as the development of malignant tumors in different organs.

Synchronous and metachronous tumors
  Tumors diagnosed within 2 months are designated as synchronous.
  Tumors diagnosed after 2 months or greater are designated as metachronous.
  In the event of both synchronous and metachronous tumors, it is referred to as synchronous/metachronous tumor.

> *Note*: The abovementioned criteria on synchronous and metachronous do not apply to cancer metastasis. Metachronous metastasis is described as metastatic lesions that are newly diagnosed after a series of examinations and/or treatments for the relevant cancer regardless of the time period between diagnosis and examinations and/or treatments.

**Familial adenomatous polyposis (FAP)
  FAP is caused by a pathological germline mutation of *APC* and is an autosomal dominant disorder primarily characterized by multiple adenomas (polyposis) of the large intestine. If left untreated, colorectal cancer will develop in almost 100% of cases (refer to clinical practice guidelines for hereditary colorectal cancer). *MUTYH*-associated polyposis caused by a pathological mutation in *MYH* and is an autosomal recessive disorder.

Lynch syndrome
  Lynch syndrome is an autosomal dominant hereditary disease mainly caused by germline mutations in mismatch repair genes. Various malignant tumors develop in conjunction with this syndrome, such as colorectal and endometrial cancers (refer to the clinical practice guidelines for hereditary colorectal cancer). The International Collaborative Group on Hereditary Non-Polyposis Colorectal Cancer (ICG-HNPCC), which plays a central role in elucidating the pathology of this syndrome, formerly referred to this condition as "hereditary non-polyposis colorectal cancer (HNPCC);" however, because the syndrome also includes tumors other than colorectal cancer, the name "Lynch syndrome" is currently recommended.

Note 4: In the narrow sense, techniques that accomplish peeling without using a snare are termed as "ESD." Techniques that implement snaring without any peeling of the submucosa after making an incision around the lesion using either an ESD knife or a snare tip are termed as "precutting EMR," and techniques that involve peeling of the submucosa after making an incision around the lesion using either an ESD knife or a snare tip with ultimate snaring are termed as "hybrid ESD."

4.2 Surgical treatment

For surgical treatment, the approach, surgical procedure, extent of lymph node dissection, anastomosis method (anastomosis form and procedure), and combined organ resection are recorded. In surgery for rectal cancer, the preservation of autonomic nerves (Page 27) is recorded.

4.2.1 Approach to the lesion

Transanal, trans-sphincter, trans-sacral, transabdominal (laparoscopic, open), and others

4.2.2 Surgical procedures

Polypectomy

Local excision

Appendectomy

Ileocecal resection

Partial colectomy

Right hemicolectomy

Left hemicolectomy

Sigmoidectomy

Subtotal colectomy

Total colectomy

Proctocolectomy

High anterior resection

Low anterior resection

Ultra-low anterior resection

Intersphincteric resection

Hartmann procedure

Abdominoperineal resection

Total pelvic exenteration

Other types of colectomy

Bypass surgery

Colostomy, ileostomy

Exploratory laparotomy

Other palliative procedures

> *Note 1*: Surgical polypectomy is a surgical method used to resect polyps at the base.
> *Note 2*: Local excision is divided into submucosal and full-thickness resections.
> *Note 3*: Colectomy other than ileocecal resection, right hemicolectomy, left hemicolectomy, sigmoid colectomy, subtotal colectomy, and total colectomy are partial colectomies.
> *Note 4*: In partial colectomy, the part of the resected colon is specified in parentheses, *e.g.*, partial colectomy (ascending colon) or partial colectomy (transverse colon).
> *Note 5*: High and low anterior resections are classified by the height of the resection line relative to the level of the peritoneal reflection.
> *Note 6*: Ultra-low anterior resection is a surgical method performed via a transabdominal approach to remove the rectum en bloc near the attachment point at the puborectal muscle (either proximal or distal side); anastomosis of the proximal side of the intestinal tract and anal canal is performed.
> *Note 7*: Intersphincteric resection (ISR) is a surgical method that involves both the transabdominal and anal approaches. It involves surgical dissection between the inner and outer sphincter, resecting the rectum en bloc together with the internal anal sphincter within the anatomical anal duct from directly above the dentate line to the intersphincteric groove, and anastomosing transanally the distal end of the sigmoid colon and the anus.
> *Note 8*: Surgical methods for treating familial adenomatous polyposis include total colectomy with ileostomy, total colectomy with ileal pouch-anal canal anastomosis (IACA), total colectomy with ileal pouch-anal anastomosis(IAA), and total colectomy with ileorectal anastomosis(IRA).

4.2.3 Lymph node dissection

4.2.3.1 Extent of lymph node dissection (D)

DX: Extent of lymph node dissection cannot be assessed

D0: Incomplete pericolic/perirectal lymph node dissection

D1: Complete pericolic/perirectal lymph node dissection

D2: Complete pericolic/perirectal and intermediate lymph node dissection

D3: Pericolic/perirectal, intermediate, and main lymph nodes are dissected

> *Note 1*: For lower rectal cancers or cancers infiltrates into the lower rectum, the extent of lateral lymph node dissection (LD) should be determined as described below and be separately recorded from the extent of dissection of the perirectal intermediate or main lymph nodes along the inferior mesenteric artery (D).
> *Note 2*: The inguinal lymph nodes (292) in rectal-type anal canal adenocarcinoma are regarded as "intermediate lymph nodes."
> *Note 3*: The extent of lymph node dissection does not apply to anal squamous cell carcinomas and

cancers arising from the anal gland and anal fistula.

4.2.3.2 Extent of lateral lymph node dissection (LD)

The extent of LD is classified as follows:

LDX: Extent of LD cannot be assessed.

LD0: LD is not performed

LD1: LD does not satisfy LD2

LD2: Dissection of 263D, 263 P, and 283 is performed

LD3: Dissection of all lateral lymph nodes is performed

Note 1: Lateral lymph nodes are 263D, 263P, 283, 273, 293, 260, 270, and 280 (Pages 44-46).

Note 2: If the extent of dissection is different on the left and right sides, then each side should be separately described and annotated using "rt-LD number" for the right and "lt-LD number" for the left.

Examples:

Right side dissections are 263D, 263P, 283, 273, 293, and 260, and left side dissections are 263D, 263P, and 283, with 270 and 280 also dissected: LD2 (rt-3/lt-2)

263D, 263P, and 283 are dissected on both left and right sides: LD2

263D, 263P, and 283 are dissected on the right side with no dissections on the left side: LD1 (rt-2/lt-0)

Note 3: For lower rectal cancers or cancer infiltrates into the lower rectum, the extent of lymph node dissection along the intestine and feeding artery (D) and the extent of LD should also be noted.

Example:

The extent of lymph node dissection along the intestine and feeding artery is D3, and the extent of LD is LD2: D3LD2.

4.2.4 Anastomosis

4.2.4.1 Types of anastomosis

End-to-end anastomosis

Side-to-end anastomosis

End-to-side anastomosis

Side-to-side anastomosis

Functional end-to-end anastomosis

Note: When an ileal or colonic pouch is constructed, it is recorded.

4.2.4.2 Methods of anastomosis
Hand-sewn anastomosis
Stapled anastomosis
Single stapling anastomosis
Double stapling anastomosis
Functional end-to-end anastomosis

4.2.5 Combined resection of adjacent organs and structures
All organs or structures resected due to cancer invasion/metastasis are recorded.

> *Note*: For combined organ resection, whether the organ is completely or partially resected should be recorded.

4.2.6 Preservation of autonomic nerves (AN) (Fig. 7)
ANX: Preservation of autonomic nerves cannot be assessed
AN0: All autonomic nerves are removed
AN1: Pelvic plexus on one side is preserved, and pelvic plexus on the other side and superior hypogastric plexus are removed
AN2: Pelvic plexuses on both sides are preserved, and superior hypogastric plexus is removed.
AN3: Pelvic plexus on one side and superior hypogastric plexus are preserved, and pelvic plexus on the other side is removed
AN4: All autonomic nerves are preserved

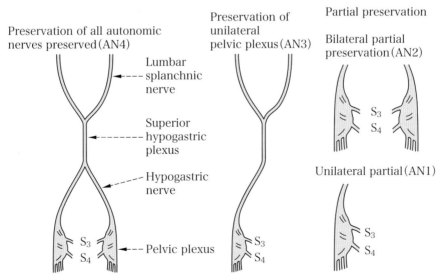

Fig. 7 Preservation of autonomic nerves

Note 1: AN involved in surgery for rectal cancer include the lumbar splanchnic nerve, superior hypogastric plexus, hypogastric nerve (sympathetic nerve), pelvic splanchnic nerve (parasympathetic nerve), pelvic plexus, and visceral branch arising from the pelvic plexus.

Note 2: In AN1 and AN3, the side of the autonomic nerves preserved is recorded. *e.g.*, AN3 rt, AN1 lt

Note 3: When partial preservation of pelvic plexus is performed, it is recorded. *e.g.*, resection of the 3rd pelvic splanchnic nerve (S3).

5 Assessment of cancer involvement at resected margin, residual tumor, and curability

5.1 Cancer involvement at resection margins

Tumor invasion in the resected margin is confirmed by histological examination.

5.1.1 Specimens obtained by endoscopic resection

5.1.1.1 Horizontal margin (lateral/mucosal margin) (HM)

HMX: Tumor involvement of the lateral margin cannot be assessed

HM0: No tumor identified at the lateral margin

HM1: Tumor identified at the lateral margin

Note 1: In HM0, the margin of clearance is measured and recorded.

Note 2: When adenoma gland alone extends to the margin in a lesion that contains both carcinoma and adenoma component, it should be recorded as HM0 (adenoma component positive).

Note 3: Specify the margin even when the lesion comprises an adenoma alone.

5.1.1.2 Vertical margin (deep/intramural margin) (VM)

VMX: Tumor involvement of the deep margin cannot be assessed

VM0: No tumor identified at the deep margin

VM1: Tumor identified at the deep margin

Note 1: In VM0, the margin of clearance is measured and recorded.

Note 2: Occurrences of local recurrence were reported in tumors with the margin clearance $<500\,\mu$m.

5.1.2 Specimens obtained by surgical resection
5.1.2.1 Proximal margin (PM)
PMX: Tumor involvement of the proximal margin cannot be assessed
PM0: No tumor identified at the proximal margin
PM1: Tumor identified at the proximal margin

5.1.2.2 Distal margin (DM)
DMX: Tumor involvement of the distal margin cannot be assessed
DM0: No tumor identified at the distal margin
DM1: Tumor identified at the distal margin

5.1.2.3 Radial margin (circumferential resection margin) (RM)
RMX: Tumor involvement of the radial margin cannot be assessed
RM0: No tumor identified at the radial margin
RM1: Tumor identified at the radial margin

Note 1: In PM0, DM0 and RM0, the distance of proximal, distal, and radial margins of clearance are measured and recorded.
Note 2: The tumor is described as HRM0 when not exposed to the cut surface of the liver and as HRM1 when exposed.

5.2 Residual tumor
5.2.1 Residual tumor following endoscopic treatment (ER)
ERX: HMX or VMX
ER0: HM0 and VM0
ER1: HM1 and/or HM1
 ER1a: HM1, VM0
 ER1b: HM0, VM1, or HM1, VM1
ER2: Macroscopic residual tumor

Note 1: Residual tumor following endoscopic treatment is histologically classified as ERX–ER1.
Note 2: Resection with a macroscopic residual tumor is defined as ER2.

5.2.2 Residual tumor following surgical treatment (R)
RX: Presence of residual tumor cannot be assessed.
R0: No residual tumor
R1: Microscopic residual tumor at resection lines or planes
R2: Macroscopic residual tumor

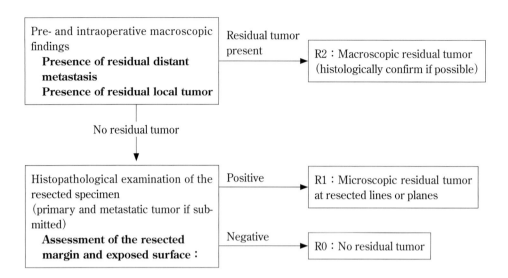

Note 1: In the event of distant metastasis (hepatic metastasis, pulmonary metastasis, and peritoneal dissemination), residual tumor is assessed for both primary tumor and distant metastasis lesions, and the greater degree of residual tumor is recorded as the final R; for example, even when the residual tumor after the primary tumor resection is R0, if the residual tumor after metastatic liver tumor resection is R1, then the final R is recorded as R1.

Note 2: In the event of the two-stage resection of distant metastasis in a Stage IV tumor, residual tumor of the primary tumor and distant metastatic tumor in the first and second stages of surgery are comprehensively assessed; for example, with synchronous pulmonary metastasis, when the primary tumor margin in the first stage of surgery is R0 (R2 in assessment of the first stage of surgery) and the margin of the pulmonary metastatic tumor in the second stage of surgery is R1, the final R is recorded as R1.

5.3 Curability

Curability with surgical treatment (Cur)

Curability X (CurX): Curability cannot be evaluated

Curability A (CurA): No distant metastasis (M0), and no residual tumor at both proximal/distal and radial margins (PM0, DM0, and RM0)

Curability B (CurB): Not corresponding to Curability A or C

Curability C (CurC): Macroscopic residual tumor

Note 1: Curability in surgical treatment is comprehensively assessed on the basis of clinical, surgical, and pathological findings.

Note 2: Excluding Tis cancers, designate the curability as unclear (CurX) for local resections without lymph node dissection.

6 Chemotherapy and radiotherapy

6.1 Chemotherapy documentation

Name of regimen used

Duration (start date and completed date of administration)

Reason for the discontinuation of administration (completion, disease progression, adverse events, refusal, etc.)

Time relationship with surgery when used in combination with surgery (prior to surgery in resectable cases, conversion in unresectable cases, and postoperative adjuvant therapy)

Indicator of the general condition [performance status (PS)] is sequentially recorded.

Response to chemotherapy is evaluated according to the Response Evaluation Criteria in Solid Tumors (RECIST), and adverse events are evaluated according to the Common Terminology Criteria for Adverse Events (CTCAE) (Pages 58, 59).

6.2 Radiotherapy documentation

6.2.1 Aims of radiotherapy

Radical, adjuvant (preoperative, intraoperative, postoperative, and combination), palliative

6.2.2 Methods of radiotherapy

Equipment (source)

Radiation quality

Energy

Radiation technique: fixed radiation, moving beam radiation, etc.

Number of beams

Treatment position

Field size

Dose per fraction (Gy)

Fractionation: number of fractions per day and per week

Treatment period

Total dose (Gy)

Whether concomitant therapy (chemotherapy, etc.) was performed and the details of it, if any

6.2.3 Radiation field

7 Evaluation of resected specimens

7.1 Macroscopic findings
7.1.1 Tumor location (Page 7)
7.1.2 Macroscopic types (Page 10)
7.1.3 Size (Page 10)
7.1.3.1 Tumor size
7.1.3.2 Size of the intramucosal component of the tumor
7.1.3.3 Size of the ulcerated area
7.1.4 Proportion of the tumor in relation to the circumference of the bowel (Page 10)
7.1.5 Distance from the lesion to the resection margin (Page 28)
7.1.6 Extent and properties of invasion and metastasis
7.1.7 Depth of tumor invasion (Page 12)
7.1.8 Lymph node metastasis and location (Page 13)

7.2 Histological findings
7.2.1 Histological types (Page 62)

A Colon and rectum

1 Benign epithelial tumors

  1.1 Adenoma

    1.1.1 Tubular adenoma

    1.1.2 Tubulovillous adenoma

    1.1.3 Villous adenoma

    1.1.4 Traditional serrated adenoma

2 Malignant epithelial tumors

  2.1 Adenocarcinoma

    2.1.1 Papillary adenocarcinoma (pap)

    2.1.2 Tubular adenocarcinoma (tub)

      2.1.2.2 Well differentiated type (tub1)

      2.1.2.2 Moderately differentiated type (tub2)

    2.1.3 Poorly differentiated adenocarcinoma (por)

      2.1.3.1 Solid type (por1)

      2.1.3.2 Non-solid type (por2)

    2.1.4 Mucinous adenocarcinoma (muc)

    2.1.5 Signet-ring cell carcinoma (sig)

    2.1.6 Medullary carcinoma (med)

2.2 Adenosquamous carcinoma (asc)

   2.3 Squamous cell carcinoma (scc)

   2.4 Carcinoid tumor

   2.5 Endocrine cell carcinoma

   2.6 Miscellaneous histological types of malignant epithelial tumors

3 Non-epithelial tumors

   3.1 Myogenic tumor

   3.2 Neurogenic tumor

   3.3 GIST (Gastrointestinal stromal tumor)

   3.4 Lipoma and lipomatosis

   3.5 Vascular tumor

   3.6 Miscellaneous tumor

4 Lymphoma

   4.1 B-cell lymphoma

      4.1.1 Mucosa-associated lymphoid tissue (MALT) lymphoma

      4.1.2 Follicular lymphoma

      4.1.3 Mantle cell lymphoma

      4.1.4 Diffuse large B-cell lymphoma

      4.1.5 Burkitt's lymphoma

      4.1.6 Others

   4.2 T-cell lymphoma

   4.3 Hodgkin's lymphoma

5 Unclassified tumors

6 Metastatic tumors

7 Tumor-like lesions

   7.1 Hyperplastic nodule

   7.2 Hyperplastic (metaplastic) polyp

   7.3 Sessile serrated adenoma/polyp (SSA/P)

   7.4 Juvenile polyp

   7.5 Inflammatory polyp and polyposis

   7.6 Inflammatory fibroid polyp

   7.7 Inflammatory myoglandular polyp

   7.8 Hamartomatous polyp

   7.9 Mucosal prolapse syndrome

   7.10 Cap polyposis

   7.11 Benign lymphoid polyp

7.12 Endometriosis
7.13 Others (Heterotopic gastric mucosa, elastofibromatous polyp, colonic muco-submucosal elongated polyp, etc.)

8 Hereditary tumors and gastrointestinal polyposis
   8.1 Familial adenomatous polyposis
   8.2 Lynch syndrome
   8.3 Peutz-Jeghers syndrome
   8.4 Serrated polyposis/hyperplastic polyposis
   8.5 Cronkhite-Canada syndrome, Cronkhite-Canada polyp
   8.6 Juvenile polyposis
   8.7 Cowden syndrome, phosphate and tensin homolog (PTEN) hamartoma tumor syndrome
   8.8 Others

B Vermiform appendix
1 Benign epithelial neoplasia
2 Low-grade appendiceal mucinous neoplasm
3 Malignant epithelial neoplasia
   3.1 Adenocarcinoma
   3.2 Goblet cell carcinoid
   3.3 Carcinoid tumor
4 Mesenchymal tumor
5 Malignant lymphoma
6 Tumor-like lesions
7 Others

C Anal canal (including perianal skin)
1 Benign epithelial neoplasia
   1.1 Adenoma
   1.2 Serrated lesion
   1.3 Condyloma acuminatum
   1.4 Squamous cell papilloma
   1.5 Hidradenoma papilliferum
   1.6 Others
2 Squamous intraepithelial neoplasia
   2.1 Low-grade intraepithelial neoplasia
   2.2 High-grade intraepithelial neoplasia

2.3 Carcinoma in situ
   2.4 Bowen's disease
   2.5 Others
3 Malignant epithelial tumors
   3.1 Adenocarcinoma
      3.1.1 Rectal-type adenocarcinoma
      3.1.2 Extramucosal (fistula-associated, perianal) adenocarcinoma
   3.2 Squamous cell carcinoma
   3.3 Adenosquamous carcinoma
   3.4 Carcinoid tumor
   3.5 Endocrine cell carcinoma
   3.6 Others
4 Malignant melanoma
5 Extramammary Paget's disease
6 Mesenchymal neoplasia
7 Malignant lymphoma
8 Tumor-like lesion
9 Others

7.2.2 Infiltration pattern (INF)

The most predominant invasion growth types at the leading front of tumor are classified into the following 3 types:

   INFa (expansive type): The tumor shows expansive growth and there is a distinct boundary between the tumor and the surrounding tissue.
   INFb (intermediate type): Intermediate between INF a and INF c.
   INFc (infiltrative type): The tumor exhibits infiltrative growth and the boundary with the surrounding normal tissue is indistinct.

   Note 1: Cancers that have grown to T1 or further are recorded.
   Note 2: Judgement is made based on images aquired using either a pathology image of loupe device or by low magnification.

7.2.3 Lymphovascular invasion
7.2.3.1 Lymphatic invasion (Ly) (Page 82, Fig. 23)

Lymphatic invasion is the invasion of tumor cells into the lymphatic vessels.
   LyX: Lymphatic invasion cannot be assessed.
   Ly0: No lymphatic invasion

Ly1: Lymphatic invasion identified.
 Ly1a: Minimal lymphatic invasion.
 Ly1b: Moderate lymphatic invasion.
 Ly1c: Severe lymphatic invasion.

7.2.3.2 Venous invasion (V) (Page 82, Fig. 24)

Venous invasion is the invasion of tumor cells into the blood vessels.
 VX: Venous invasion cannot be assessed.
 V0: No venous invasion.
 V1: Microscopic venous invasion.
  V1a: Minimal venous invasion.
  V1b: Moderate venous invasion.
  V1c: Severe venous invasion.
 V2: Macroscopic venous invasion

Note 1: Invasion of the vascular system is assessed with pathological specimens prepared from the section of tumor at the largest tumor diameter.
Note 2: When immunostaining is used to examine for lymphatic invasion, it should be stated. *e.g.*, Ly1a (D2-40)
Note 3: When elastic fiber staining is used to examine for venous invasion, it should be stated. *e.g.*, V1a (VB) with Victoria blue staining, V1b (EVG) with Elastica van Gieson staining.
Note 4: When vascular invasion is present but it is difficult to judge whether this is lymphatic invasion or venous invasion, designate it as Ly/V.
Note 5: The level of the deepest vascular invasion should be recorded. *e.g.*, V1a (SS) (EVG)
Note 6: When a tumor has an elastic plate confirmed at one-half or more of its circumference, it is considered as "V," and when D2-40-positive endothelial cells are confirmed at one-half or more of its circumference, it is considered as "Ly". Using this method, inconsistencies among individuals judging vascular invasions should be reduced.
Note 7: Subtyping of Ly1 and V1 is not needed for endoscopic resection specimens.

7.2.4 Tumor budding (BD)

"Tumor budding" is defined as a cancer cell nest consisting of one or fewer than five cells that infiltrates the interstitium at the invasive margin of the cancer.

On selecting the region where tumor budding is the greatest, the front of the tumor growth is observed at 200× magnification to count the number of tumor buds (Page 83, Fig. 25).
 BDX: Budding cannot be assessed.
 BD1: 0-4 buds
 BD2: 5-9 buds

BD3: 10 or more buds

> *Note*: BD should be described in case of T1 cancer. In the cancers of T2 or greater, describe if possible.

7.2.5 Extramural cancer deposits without lymph node structure (EX) (page 38)

Extramural cancer deposits with no lymph node structure (EX) within the regional lymph node area should be recorded. EX includes localized lesions comprising lymphatic invasion, venous invasion, perineural invasion (vascular/perineural invasion lesions), and other lesions (tumor nodule: ND) (Page 83, Fig. 26).

> *Note 1*: All tumor deposits located in the extramural fatty tissue are regarded as EX in tumors in which continuous spread was confined within the SM or MP. For tumors that directly penetrate the MP, tumor deposits located ≥5 mm from the leading edge of the primary tumor are designated as EX.
>
> *Note 2*: ND is treated as lymph node metastasis (Page 17).
>
> *Note 3*: ND involving veins and/or neural fascicles at their growing front should be designated as ND(V+), ND(Pn+), or ND(V&Pn+) because these are associated with an extremely poor prognosis (Page 83, Fig. 27).
>
> *Note 4*: When localized foci of lymphovascular or perineural invasion are identified, the number of foci should be described in parentheses per relevant lymph node station. *e.g.*, if one focus of each lymphatic and venous invasion is identified in station 201, then it would be described as #201: Ly (1), V (1).

7.2.6 Perineural invasion (Pn)

PnX: Perineural invasion cannot be assessed.

Pn0: No perineural invasion.

Pn1: Presence of perineural invasion.

 Pn1a: Intramural perineural invasion only.

 Pn1b: Extramural perineural invasion.

> *Note 1*: A distinctive pattern of horizontal spread in a form to replace the myenteric (Auerbach's) plexus can be regarded as intramural perineural invasion, irrespective of the confirmation of perineural invasion (Page 84, Fig. 28).
>
> *Note 2*: Extramural perineural invasion was histological finding of tumor cells invading or spreading a long nerve fascicles external to the MP. Extramural perineural invasion exists as an isolated lesion (Page 84, Fig. 29) or within the body of the primary tumor (Page 85, Fig. 30). In diagnosing the latter, emphasis is placed on findings of tumor nests in direct contact with nerve fascicle without being intervened by connective tissue.

38   I. Guidelines for classification

7.3 Histological criteria for the assessment of response to chemotherapy/radiotherapy

Grade 0 (No effect): No tumor cell necrosis or degeneration in response to treatment is observed.

Grade 1 (Mild effect)

  (a) Minimal effect: Tumor cell necrosis or degeneration is present in less than one-third of the entire lesion.

  (b) Mild effect: Tumor cell necrosis, degeneration, and/or lytic change is present in more than one-third but less than two-third of the entire lesion.

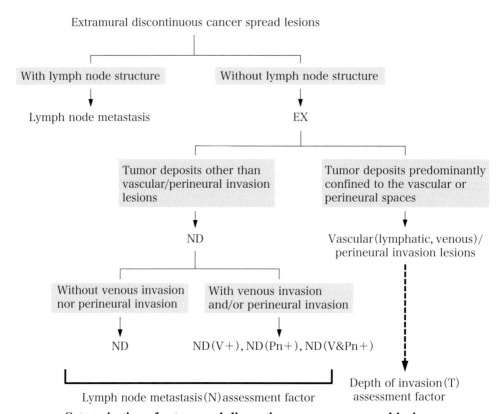

Categorization of extramural discontinuous cancer spread lesions

Grade 2 (Moderate effect): Prominent tumor cell necrosis, degeneration, lytic change, and/or disappearance is present in more than two-third of the entire lesion, but viable tumor cells remain.

Grade 3 (Marked effect): Necrosis and/or lytic change is present throughout the entire lesion and is replaced by fibrosis with or without granulomatous change. No viable tumor cells are observed.

> *Note*: Assessment is performed on pathological specimens as many as possible, including those prepared from the section of whole tumor at its largest diameter.

7.4 Histological assessment of biopsy specimens (Group classification) (Page 74)

Group X: Inadequate material for histological diagnosis
Group 1: Normal tissue or a non-neoplastic lesion
Group 2: Lesions in which it is difficult to determine whether the lesion is neoplastic or non-neoplastic
Group 3: Benign tumor
Group 4: Neoplastic lesion suspected of being carcinoma
Group 5: Carcinoma

7.5 Measurement of the depth of invasion

7.5.1 T1 cancer (Fig. 8; Page 56, Fig. 18)

Irrespective of the macroscopic type, when it is possible to identify or estimate the location of the muscularis mucosa, the depth of submucosal invasion is measured from the lower border of the muscularis mucosa (Fig. 8-1, Fig. 18-①), whereas when this is not possible, the depth of invasion is measured from the surface of the lesion (Fig. 8-2, Fig. 18-②, ③).

> *Note 1*: In this description, the phrase "possible to identify or estimate the location" indicates that there is no "deformity" caused by submucosal invasion, i.e., muscularis mucosa without disarray, dissection, rupture, or fragmentation. When a deformed muscularis mucosa is used as the baseline of measurement, the depth of submucosal invasion can be underestimated. Although it is not necessarily easy to judge whether there is a "deformity," if there is a desmoplastic reaction present around the muscularis mucosa, then it is assumed to be "deformed."
>
> *Note 2*: In pedunculated lesions with a tangled muscularis mucosa, it may not be possible to identify the muscularis mucosa to use as the baseline to measure invasion. In such instances, the depth of submucosal invasion is measured as the distance between the point of the deepest invasion and the reference line, which is defined as the neck (boundary between the tumor head and the stalk) (Fig. 18-④). Pedunculated lesions with a tangled muscula-

40   I. Guidelines for classification

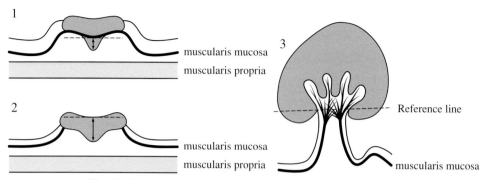

Fig. 8   Measurement of the depth of invasion in T1 cancers

ris mucosa, in which invasion is limited to within the head, are defined as "head invasion" (Fig. 8-3, Fig. 18-⑤).

Note 3: Differentiation is required for the findings of submucosal infiltration of tubular adenoma glands, i. e, pseudocarcinomatous invasion (submucosal misplacement and submucosal pseudoinvasion) (Page 88, Fig. 37).

7.5.2 Tumor invading beyond the MP in sites without the serosa

The depth of extramural invasion is measured at the deepest part of the tumor.
The distance is measured at the site of continuous spread of the tumor.

Note 1: Lymphatic/venous/perineural invasion, that is not contiguous from the main lesion, are not included in the measurement site.

Note 2: When the MP is preserved, the distance from the lower border of the MP to the deepest part of the extramural invasion is measured.

Note 3: When the lower border of the MP is not entirely indentifiable, the distance from the uppermost limit of the lower border of the MP where to the deepest part of the extramural invasion is measured. When there is a right and left difference at the ruptured edge of the MP, the distance from the lower edge of break point of the MP closest to the tumor surface to the deepest part of the extramural invasion is measured.

8 Treatment outcome record

Following data are recorded for statistical analysis:

8.1 Number of patients

Total number of outpatients with colorectal cancer
Total number of inpatients with colorectal cancer

8.2 Multiple colorectal cancers, multiple primary cancers (Page 22)

8.3 Modalities of treatment and adjuvant therapy
Endoscopic treatment
Surgical treatment
Chemotherapy
Radiotherapy
Other non-operative treatment
No treatment

> *Note*: Refer to Section 4.2. Surgical treatment (Page 24) when documenting surgical procedures.

8.4 Total number of colorectal cancer cases with treatment, and the number and rate of cases by treatment types
The number of cases and the proportion by treatment methods and types are described.

8.4.1 Resection rate
Resection rate = number of patients who underwent surgical resection of tumors/total number of surgical patients

Number and proportion of patients who underwent surgical resection of tumors with respect to each curability (A, B, and C).

> *Note*: The number of resection surgeries includes polypectomy and local excision in addition to intestinal resection.

8.4.2 Endoscopic treatment
Patients treated by endoscopic procedure alone are distinguished from those who underwent surgical resection.

8.4.3 Chemotherapy and radiotherapy
The number and proportion of patients who underwent chemotherapy and radiation therapy are recorded according to the RECIST outcome.

8.5 Number and rate of operative mortality

> *Note 1*: Operative mortality is defined as death within 30 days after surgery irrespective of whether the patient was in the hospital or discharged.

Note 2: Rate of operative mortality is defined as the ratio of the number of operative death to the total number of patients who underwent surgery.

8.6 Number and rate of hospital mortality following surgery

Note 1: Hospital mortality is defined as death while in hospital following any surgical treatment.
Note 2: The rate of hospital mortality is defined as the ratio of the number of hospital deaths to the total number of patients who underwent surgical treatment.

8.7 Survival analysis

Following data are recorded for survival analysis:

8.7.1 Survival

Alive: The most recent date of follow-up is recorded.
Dead: The date of death is recorded.
Unknown (lost to follow-up): The final date of follow-up is recorded.
Cause of death
  Treatment-related death
  Death due to colorectal cancer
  Death due to other malignancy: the name of the malignancy is recorded
  Death due to other disease: the name of the disease is recorded (not including deaths from other malignant tumors).
  Death due to accidents, including suicide
  Death due to unknown cause.

8.7.2 Recurrence/metastasis; site(s) and mode

Presence or absence of recurrence
Date when recurrence is confirmed
Methods for confirming recurrence
Site(s) and mode of recurrence
  Note: Site(s) and mode of each recurrence are recorded in the order in which they were confirmed.
  Local recurrence
    Anastomotic recurrence
    Recurrence in regional lymph nodes
    Other type of local recurrence

Lymph node metastasis (recurrence in non-regional lymph nodes)

Liver metastasis

Lung metastasis

Hematogenous metastasis (other than liver and lung metastases)

Peritoneal metastasis

Recurrence at unspecified sites

Note: Sites of recurrence are recorded using abbreviation demonstrated 3.2.2 Distant metastasis (M) (Pages 17–18).

8.7.3 Survival analysis method

Following data are recorded for statistical analysis:

Target population (i.e., patients who underwent endoscopic treatment, surgical treatment, etc.)

Methods of estimating survival

    Actuarial survival rate

        Direct method

        Cumulative survival rate: Life-table method, Kaplan-Meier method

    Relative survival rate

Event classification

    All deaths, colorectal tumor deaths (primary tumor death), recurrence, secondary cancer, progression, and treatment discontinuation (Page 58)

Test of significance for survival rates

Proportion of patients lost in follow-up

Supplement: Lymph node groups and station number

Table 4 Lymph node groups and station number

	Superior mesenteric artery	Inferior mesenteric artery	Iliac artery
Pericolic/perirectal lymph nodes	Lymph nodes along the marginal arteries and near the bowel wall · Pericolic lymph nodes (201, 211, 221)	Lymph nodes along the marginal arteries, near the bowel wall, and along the terminal sigmoid artery · Pericolic lymph nodes (231, 241: 241-1, 241-2, 241-t) Lymph nodes along the superior rectal artery · Perirectal lymph nodes (251)	Lymph nodes medial to the pelvic nerve plexus along the middle rectal artery. · Perirectal lymph nodes (251)
Intermediate lymph nodes	Lymph nodes along the ileocolic, right colic, and middle colic arteries. · Ileocolic nodes (202) · Right colic nodes (212) · Right middle colic nodes (222-rt) · Left middle colic nodes (222-lt)	Lymph nodes along the left colic and sigmoid arteries and the inferior mesenteric artery between the origin of the left colic artery of the terminal sigmoid artery · Left colic nodes (232) · Sigmoid colic nodes (242: 242-1, 242-2) · Inferior mesenteric trunk nodes (252)	
Main lymph nodes	Lymph nodes at the origin of the ileocolic, right colic, and middle colic arteries · Ileocolic root nodes (203) · Right colic root nodes (213) · Middle colic root nodes (223)	Lymph nodes along the inferior mesenteric artery from the origin of the inferior mesenteric artery to that of the left colic artery · Inferior mesenteric root nodes (253)	

Supplement: Lymph node groups and station number

Lateral lymph nodes		Lymph nodes along the internal iliac arteries and along the obturator vessels and nerves ・Proximal internal iliac nodes (263P) ・Distal internal iliac nodes (263D) ・Obturator nodes (283) Lymph nodes along the common iliac external iliac, and median sacral arteries ・Common iliac nodes (273) ・External iliac nodes (293) ・Lateral sacral nodes (260) ・Median sacral nodes (270) ・Aortic bifurcation nodes (280) ・Inguinal nodes (292)
Downward lymph nodes		
Lymph nodes proximal to the main lymph nodes	Lymph nodes at the origin of the superior mesenteric artery and along the aorta ・Superior mesenteric arterial root nodes (214) ・Para-aortic nodes (216)	Lymph nodes along the aorta ・Para-aortic nodes (216)
Other lymph nodes	・Sub-pyloric nodes (206) ・Gastroepiploic nodes (204) ・Splenic hilar nodes (210)	

Note 1: The sigmoid artery commonly comprises the first, second, and terminal arteries, with pericolic lymph nodes recorded as 241-1, 242-2, and 241-t, respectively, and intermediate lymph nodes recorded as 242-1 and 242-2.

Note 2: Iliac arterial lymph nodes are recorded according to whether they are to the left or right (right=rt and left=lt), *e.g.*, right distal internal iliac lymph nodes are recorded as rt263D.

Note 3: In anal cancer, 292 is treated as intermediate lymph nodes.

46   I. Guidelines for classification

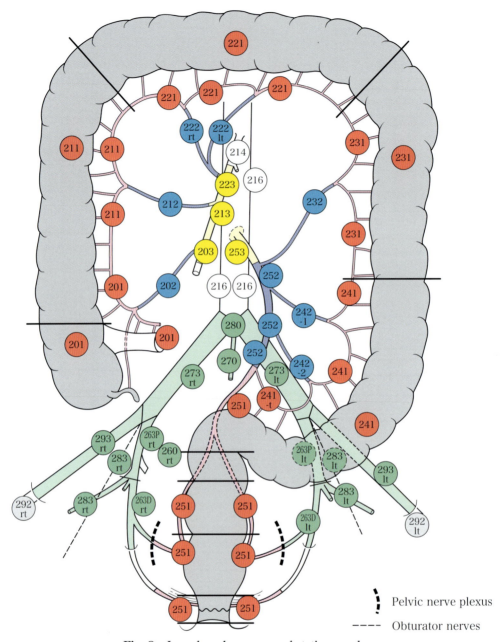

Fig. 9   Lymph node groups and station numbers
Red: Pericolic/perirectal lymph nodes
Blue: Intermediate lymph nodes
Yellow: Main lymph nodes
Green: Lateral lymph nodes
Gray: Downward lymph nodes
White: Lymph nodes proximal to the main lymph nodes

Supplementary Reference of Macroscopic Types

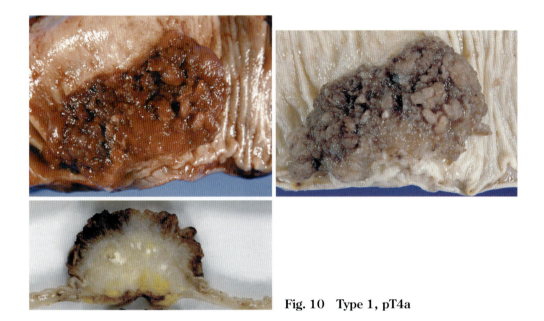

Fig. 10 Type 1, pT4a

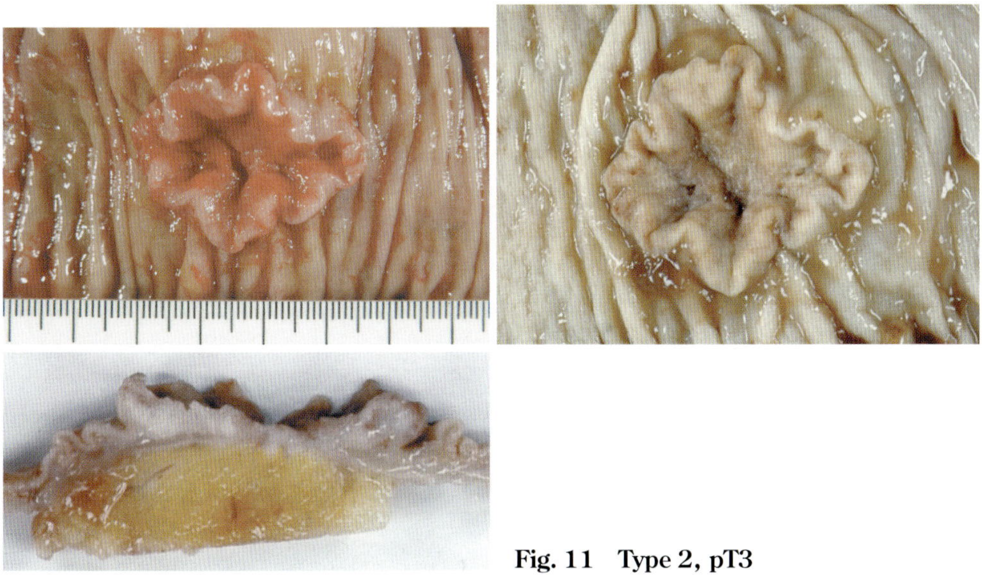

Fig. 11 Type 2, pT3

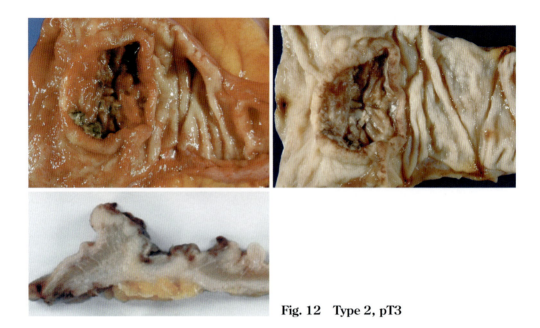

Fig. 12 Type 2, pT3

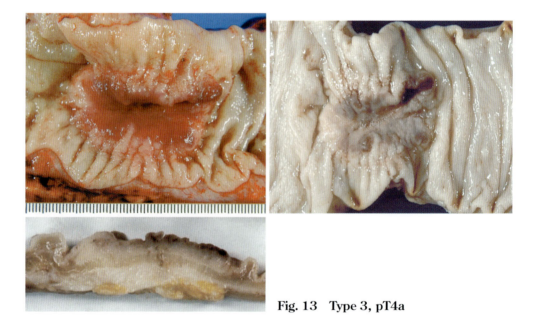

Fig. 13 Type 3, pT4a

Supplementary Reference of Macroscopic Types 49

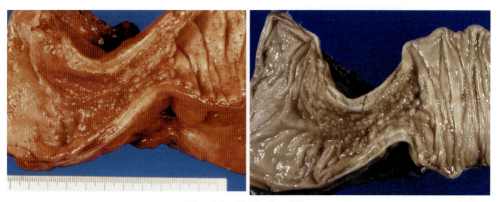

Fig. 14 Type 4, pT4a

50   I. Guidelines for classification

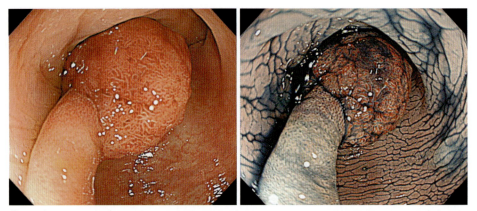

① 0-Ip (pedunculated): Polyp with stalk. This must be differentiated from a pseudopeduncle that appears like a stalk made from mucosa at the site of adhesion being pulled.

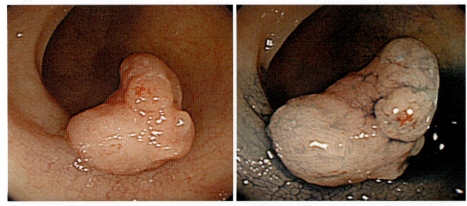

② 0-Isp (semi-pedunculated): Spherical polyp. Part of the lesion is attached to the bowel wall.

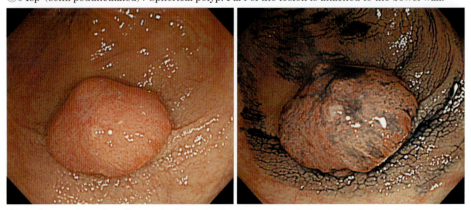

③ 0-Is (non-pedunculated): Hemispherical polyp. Base of the lesion is attached to the bowel wall.

Fig. 15 Subtypes of macroscopic type 0

Supplementary Reference of Macroscopic Types 51

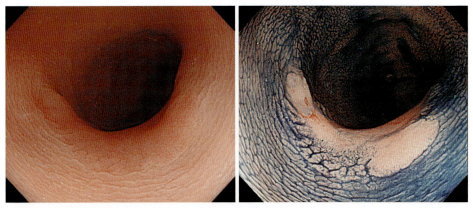

④0-IIa (superficial elevated type): Flat elevated lesion with a smooth surface.

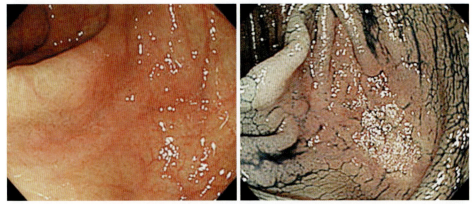

⑤0-IIb (superficial flat type): The lesion has a smooth surface and is almost at the same height as the mucosa.

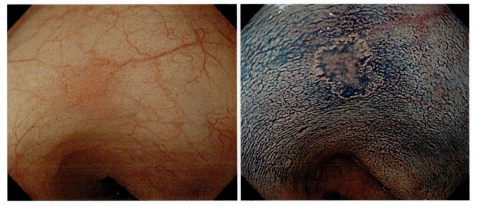

⑥0-IIc (superficial depressed type): Depressed lesion. Horizontal level of the lesion is lower than that of the mucosal surface, and its margin is often slightly elevated by reactive changes.

Fig. 15 Subtypes of macroscopic type 0 (continued)

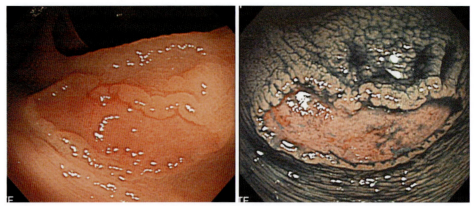

⑦ 0-IIc+IIa (complex type): Depressed lesion with elevated margin. Horizontal level of the depressed part of the lesion is lower than that of the mucosal surface, and its elevated margin formed by reactive changes is conspicuous.

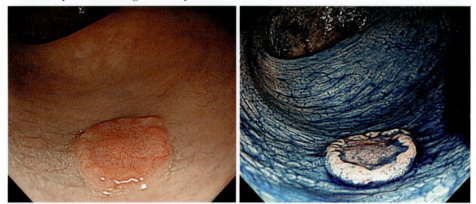

⑧ 0-IIa+IIc (complex type): Flat elevated lesion with a depressed surface higher than the mucosa. "Upstairs depression" and "downstairs depression" are often used for the depressed surface of 0-IIa+IIc and 0-IIc+IIa, respectively, as metaphorical expressions.

Fig. 15 Subtypes of macroscopic type 0 (continued)

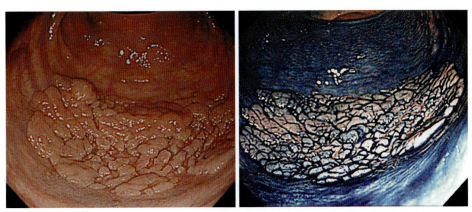

①LST-G homogeneous type: Laterally growing lesion forming similarly sized granular aggregates. Macroscopic type of the lesions is 0-IIa.

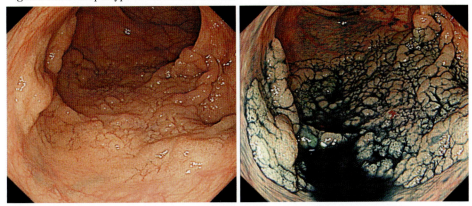

②LST-G mixed nodular type: Lesion consists of aggregated uniform sized granules and some slightly large nodules that grow horizontally. Macroscopic type is 0-IIa+Is.

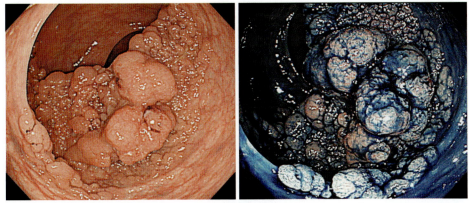

③LST-G nodular mixed type: Lesion consists of aggregated uniform sized granules and large nodules that grow horizontally. Large nodules are more prominent than uniform sized granules. Macroscopic type is 0-Is+IIa.

Fig. 16 Laterally spreading tumor (LST) subtypes

54   I. Guidelines for classification

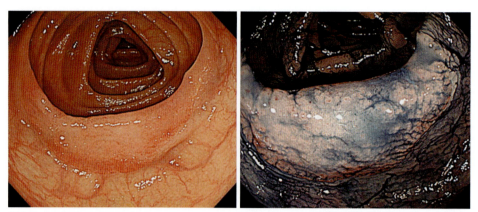

④LST-NG flat elevated type: Large flat elevated lesion extending horizontally across a semilunar fold. Macroscopic type is 0-IIa.

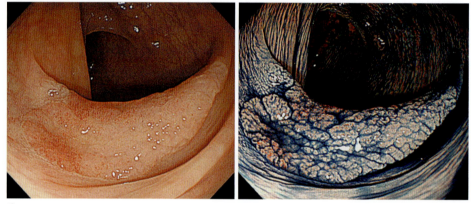

⑤LST-NG flat elevated type: Large flat elevated lesion extending horizontally across a semilunar fold. Although the illustrated lesion has hexagonal grooves, it is a flat protruded lesion as a whole, unlike LST-G. Macroscopic type is 0-IIa.

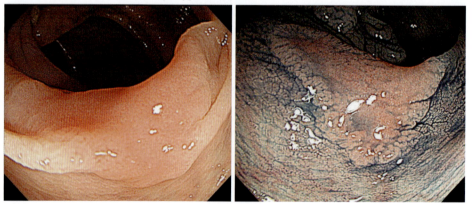

⑥LST-NG pseudodepressed type: Large flat elevated lesion with a sagging-type shallow central depression. Border of the depression cannot be shown with a single circumferential line, and the right border of the depression is obscure in the illustrated lesion. Macroscopic type is 0-IIa+IIc.

Fig. 16   Laterally spreading tumor (LST) subtypes (continued)

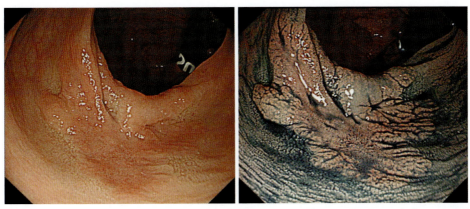

⑦LST-NG pseudodepressed type: Large flat elevated lesion with a sagging-type shallow central depression and pseudopodia-like lobulation can be seen in the margin. The oral side appears flat and elevated, whereas the anal side has a shallow depression; however, concave regions are unclear. Macroscopic observation reveals the type of the lesions to be 0-IIa+IIc.

Fig. 16 Laterally spreading tumor (LST) subtypes (continued)

Subtypes of LST	Classification in type 0	
Granular LST (LST-G)		
Homogenous	0-IIa	0-IIa
Nodular mixed	0-IIa, 0-Is+IIa, 0-IIa+Is	0-IIa+Is
Non-granular LST (LST-NG)		
Flat elevated	0-IIa	0-IIa
Pseudodepressed	0-IIa+IIc, 0-IIc+IIa	0-IIc+IIa

＊The term "laterally spreading tumor" (LST) refers to the lateral growth of lesions of at least 10 mm in diameter, as opposed to traditional polypoid (upward growth) or flat and depressed lesions (downward growth).

Fig. 17 Relationship between laterally spreading tumor (LST) subtype and macroscopic type

[cited from Kudo S, et al. Gastrointest Endosc, 2008: 68 (4 Suppl): S3-47]

56　I. Guidelines for classification

Supplement: Measurement of submucosal invasion distance

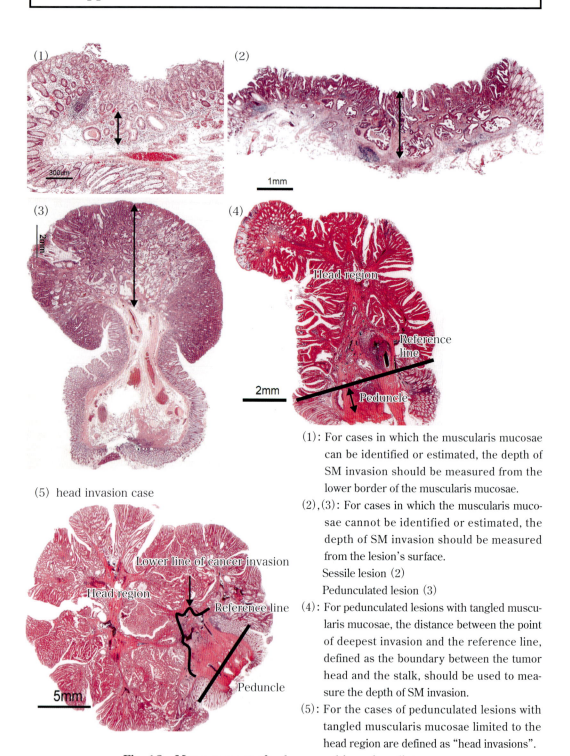

(5) head invasion case

(1): For cases in which the muscularis mucosae can be identified or estimated, the depth of SM invasion should be measured from the lower border of the muscularis mucosae.

(2),(3): For cases in which the muscularis mucosae cannot be identified or estimated, the depth of SM invasion should be measured from the lesion's surface.
Sessile lesion (2)
Pedunculated lesion (3)

(4): For pedunculated lesions with tangled muscularis mucosae, the distance between the point of deepest invasion and the reference line, defined as the boundary between the tumor head and the stalk, should be used to measure the depth of SM invasion.

(5): For the cases of pedunculated lesions with tangled muscularis mucosae limited to the head region are defined as "head invasions".

Fig. 18　Measurement of submucosal invasion distance

II. Assessment of response to chemotherapy and radiotherapy

1 Assessment of response

It is recommended to record the assessment of response in accordance with the latest version of the new guidelines for the Response Evaluation Criteria in Solid Tumors (RECIST*). However, due care should be given to the fact that the RECIST guidelines are a set of guidelines that specify standard methods of evaluating solid cancers and definitions for the objective evaluation of changes in tumor size in a clinical trial setting and are not intended for use in decision making on whether to continue treatment in routine clinical practice.

> *Japanese translation is available on the JCOG Web site
> (http://www.jcog.jp/doctor/tool/RECISTv11J_20100810.pdf).

2 Definition of efficacy endpoints

2.1 Response rate

Patients with best overall responses of either CR or PR are considered to have responded to treatment, and these are used to calculate the response rate. All patients who meet the eligibility criteria, including those assigned NE, should be included in analysis of the response rate.

2.2 Overall survival (OS), progression-free survival (PFS), relapse-free survival (RFS), disease-free survival (DFS), time to treatment failure (TTF)

Primary endpoints for efficacy other than response rate include OS, PFS, RFS, DFS, and TTF. The definitions of events in each survival period are listed below (Table 5). All eligible patients should be included in analysis. The date of registration is the starting date.

Table 5 Definition of endpoints and events

Endpoints	Events (the earliest event is counted)		
Overall survival (OS)	All-cause death		
Progression-free survival (PFS)	All-cause death	Disease progression/Relapse	
Relapse-free survival (RFS)	All-cause death	Relapse	
Disease-free survival (DFS)	All-cause death	Relapse	Secondary cancer
Time to treatment failure (TTF)	All-cause death	Disease progression/Relapse (in the event that treatment is completed)	Withdrawal of treatment

3 Documentation of adverse events

Adverse events are recorded with respect to each treatment. This includes type, incidence rate, grade, time of occurrence, duration, and reversibility of the adverse events. The assessment of adverse events should preferably be recorded according to the latest version of the Common Terminology Criteria for Adverse Events (CTCAE) http://ctep.cancer.gov/protocolDevelopment/electronic_applications/ctc.htm). The Japanese translation of the CTCAE is available on the JCOG website (http://www.jcog.jp/doctor/tool/ctcaev4.html).

III. Explanation of pathological items [Supplement: Histology Atlas]

62 III. Explanation of pathological items [Supplement: Histology Atlas]

1 Histological types

A. Colon and rectum
1 Benign epithelial tumor
1.1 Adenoma

Most adenomas in the large intestine are circumscribed elevated lesions (protruded or superficial type).

Their surface is usually granular, lobulated, or gyrus-like, but papillary or villous structure is sometimes seen.

Based on their microscopic architecture, adenomas are classified as tubular, tubulovillous, villous, or serrated.

Adenomas are classified according to their degree of atypia into low-grade (equivalent to adenomas with conventional mild and moderate atypia), high-grade (equivalent to adenomas with conventional severe atypia), and a mixture of low- and high-grade adenomas (Figs. 31-36).

> *Note*: Adenomas with replacement of the submucosa, i.e., pseudocarcinomatous invasion, should not be diagnosed as carcinomas that have invaded the submucosa (Fig. 37).

1.1.1 Tubular adenoma
Tubular adenomas mainly comprise tubular structures. In general, high proliferative activity is seen in the upper portion of the glands (Figs. 31-33).

1.1.2 Tubulovillous adenoma
Tubulovillous adenoma: an intermediate or a mixture of tubular and villous adenomas (Fig. 34).

1.1.3 Villous adenoma
Villous adenomas comprise leaf- or finger-like processes with a narrow core of lamina propria and no branching. In general, high proliferative activity is seen in the upper portion of the glands, but it may also be seen throughout their entire length (Fig. 35).

1.1.4 Traditional serrated adenoma
Serrated adenomas resemble hyperplastic polyps due to serrated morphology of the epithelium in the upper half of the duct. Nuclear swelling, pseudostratification, and mitotic figures are also visible in the surface layer, and there is a reduced number of goblet cells and eosinophilic cytoplasm (Fig. 36). Characteristic findings used to differentiate a serrated adenoma from a sessile serrated adenoma/polyp (SSA/P) and hyperplastic polyps include histological features such as ectopic crypt formation (ECF) or budding (Fig. 36, bottom figure).

2 Malignant epithelial tumors

Histological types of carcinoma of the colon and rectum can be classified as follows:

Tumors that contain more than one histological type of carcinoma are classified based on the most predominant histological type. Any other histological findings have been listed according to their dominancy (*e.g.*, tub1>pap).

> *Note*: When both carcinoma and an adenoma component are present in the same lesion, record it as "carcinoma with adenoma." Carcinoma with adenoma is classified into the following 2 types according to the proportions of the tumor occupied by the carcinoma and adenoma components:
>   a. Carcinoma in adenoma: Carcinoma with adenoma in which the carcinoma component is smaller than the adenoma component.
>   b. Carcinoma with adenoma component: Carcinoma with adenoma in which the carcinoma component is the same size or larger than the adenoma component.

2.1 Adenocarcinoma

Adenocarcinoma is characterized by malignant glandular epithelium having a tubular or papillary architecture or that producing mucin.

2.1.1 Papillary adenocarcinoma (pap)

Papillary adenocarcinomas have a papillary glandular structure comprising columnar or cuboidal cells. Carcinoma with a villous or serrated architecture is also included in this type (Fig. 38).

2.1.2 Tubular adenocarcinoma (tub)

Well differentiated tubular adenocarcinoma is characterized by distinct and large tubular structure, and moderately differentiated tubular adenocarcinoma is characterized by a medium to small tubular structures or cribriform structures.

2.1.2.1 Well differentiated type (tub1) (Figs. 39-41)
2.1.2.2 Moderately differentiated type (tub2) (Figs. 42, 43)

2.1.3 Poorly differentiated adenocarcinoma (por)

Poorly differentiated adenocarcinomas are defined as those having little tendency to form glands or tubules or those without gland and tubule formation that are positive for intracellular mucin production. The tumor displays a solid or non-solid growth pattern.

2.1.3.1 Solid type (por1) (Fig. 44)
2.1.3.2 Non-solid type (por2) (Fig. 45)

> *Note 1*: In poorly differentiated adenocarcinomas, the solid type comprises cancer cells that form a simple solid or sheet-like structure and exhibit expansive growth, whereas the non-

solid type comprises cancer cells with small glands, which form small clusters or canalicular structures, or comprises isolated cancer cells and exhibits infiltrative growth.

Note 2: Carcinoma with lymphoid stroma, characterized by marked infiltration of lymphocytes and plasma cells, is classified as non-solid type.

2.1.4 Mucinous adenocarcinoma (muc)

Mucinous adenocarcinoma comprises cells that produce substantial amount of mucin outside the cells, forming mucinous nodules or lakes. It comprises well differentiated mucinous adenocarcinoma originating from well differentiated type adenocarcinoma (papillary adenocarcinoma, well and moderately differentiated tubular adenocarcinoma) and poorly differentiated mucinous adenocarcinoma originating from poorly differentiated type adenocarcinoma (non-solid type, signet-ring cell carcinoma) (Fig. 46).

2.1.5 Signet-ring cell carcinoma (sig)

Tumor cells in signet-ring cell carcinoma are characterized by intracellular accumulation of mucin, which exhibit signet ring structures. They have little tendency to form glands or tubules (Fig. 47).

The signet-ring cells resemble intestinal goblet cells, both histochemically and electron microscopically.

2.1.6 Medullary carcinoma (med)

Medullary carcinomas are composed of eosinophilic cytoplasm and clear nucleoli with marked lymphocyte infiltration and grow in a sheet-like arrangement (Fig. 48).

2.2 Adenosquamous carcinoma (asc)

Adenosquamous carcinoma comprises a mixture of adenocarcinoma and squamous cell carcinoma. The 2 histological components may be intermingled or there may be a clear boundary between them (Fig. 49).

2.3 Squamous cell carcinoma (scc)

Squamous cell carcinoma is rare in the large intestine.

Note: Squamous cell carcinoma arising from the epithelium of the anal canal is classified as squamous cell carcinoma of the anal canal.

2.4 Carcinoid tumors (Fig. 50)

Carcinoid tumors are cancers of low-grade cells that differentiate into endocrine cells. Small, uniform, round and columnar cells show alveolar and funicular (ribbon) arrangements that occasionally display a rosette- or tubular structure-like configuration. The space between the nests is narrow with concomitant capillaries, but fibrous and fibromuscular interstices are also observed. Differentiation into endocrine cells is verified using immunostaining or other techniques, and it is necessary to discriminate these tumors from solid poorly differentiated adenocarcinomas. Although they occur deep in the mucosa, the main area of development gradually moves to the submucosa. The prevalent site of carcinoid tumors within the large intestine is ethnically specific: in the Japanese population, these occur in the lower part of the rectum and in the Western population, they occur in the appendix. These tumors are generally of low-grade malignancy.

> *Note 1*: Immunohistochemically, carcinoid tumors are mainly positive for chromogranin A, synaptophysin, and CD56 (neural cell adhesion molecule, NCAM). If carcinoid tumors are morphologically suspected, then immunostaining is strongly recommended.
> *Note 2*: Carcinoid tumor corresponds to the World Health Organization (WHO) classification for neuroendocrine tumors (NET). The WHO classification grades tumors on the basis of the number of mitoses and the Ki-67 index present (Table 6).
> *Note 3*: Adenocarcinomas have a different TNM classification (Supplementary-1, TNM classification).
> *Note 4*: According to the WHO classification, pancreatic neuroendocrine tumors are classified as per Reference (Page 66), but it is undecided whether these classification and evaluation standards apply to gastrointestinal carcinoids.
> *Note 5*: Classify goblet cell carcinoids of the appendix separately from these tumors. Refer to the section on the appendix.

2.5 Endocrine cell carcinoma (Fig. 51)

Endocrine cell carcinomas are cancers that are characterized by solid growth of highly atypical cells differentiating into endocrine cells. The tumor sizes are almost even with small or large cancer cells growing as sheets and large solid nests. Irregular funicular arrays and rosette-like structures may be observed. Considerable tumor necrosis is also present. The nucleus of these tumors is larger than that of carcinoid tumors, and a high degree of mitosis is observed. The interstices are rich with capillaries. To diagnose these tumors, it is necessary to evaluate endocrine cell differentiation using techniques such as histochemistry, electron microscopy, and immunohistochemistry. These tumors may be classified into small (small cell carcinomas) and large cell type according to the size of the predominant cancer cells. In small cell types, little cytoplasm is observed, whereas in large cell types, an abundance of cytoplasm is observed. These tumors are highly malignant.

> *Note 1*: These tumors correspond to neuroendocrine carcinomas (NECs) by the WHO classification scheme (Table 6).

Note 2: Immunohistochemically, these tumors are mainly positive for chromogranin A, synaptophysin, and neural cell adhesion molecule (NCAM, CD56). If endocrine cell carcinomas are morphologically suspected, then immunostaining is strongly recommended.

Note 3: These tumors may coexist with adenocarcinomas and, in Japan, are called "adenoendocrine cell carcinomas." According to the WHO classification scheme, cancers wherein both endocrine cell carcinoma and adenocarcinoma components occupy 30% or more of the tumor are defined as mixed adenoneuroendocrine carcinomas (MANECs).

Table 6 Relationship between the current guidelines and WHO classification

Japanese Classification of Colorectal, Appendiceal, and Anal Carcinoma (Current version)	WHO classification (2010)	Ki-67 proliferation index (%)	Mitotic index*
Carcinoid tumor	NET G1	≤2	<2
	NET G2	3–20	2–20
Endocrine cell carcinoma	NEC	>20	>20

NET=neuroendocrine tumor, NEC=neuroendocrine carcinoma, G=grade
*per 10 high power field

Reference. The WHO classification of pancreatic endocrine tumors (2017)*

Classification/grade	Ki-67 proliferation index	Mitotic index
Pancreatic neuroendocrine tumours (PanNETs)		
PanNET G1	<3%	<2
PanNET G2	3–20%	2–20
PanNET G3	>20%	>20
Pancreatic neuroendocrine carcinomas (PanNECs)		
PanNEC (G3) Small cell type/Large cell type	>20%	>20
Mixed neuroendocrine-non-neuroendocrine neoplasm (MiNEN)		

*It is undecided whether these classification and evaluation standards apply to gastrointestinal carcinoids.

2.6 Others: Miscellaneous histological types of epithelial malignant tumors

Miscellaneous carcinomas comprise choriocarcinoma, α-fetoprotein-producing adenocarcinoma, undifferentiated carcinoma, etc.

Undifferentiated carcinoma comprises small or large malignant cells forming a sheet-like or large solid structure. It lacks a glandular structure, and no mucin secretion or neuroendocrine granules are demonstrated by immunohistochemistry or other methods.

3 Non-epithelial tumors

3.1 Myogenic tumors

Myogenic tumors arise from the muscularis mucosae or the MP and may show nuclear palisading. Myogenic tumors that have low cellularity and lack mitotic figures are leiomyomas, and those that have high cellularity and numerous mitotic figures are leiomyosarcomas.

Myogenic tumors are immunostain positive for α-smooth muscle actin, muscle-specific actin and desmin, and stain negative for KIT (CD117).

3.2 Neurogenic tumor

Schwannoma is the most common neurogenic tumor, and multiple schwannomas are observed in patients with von Recklinghausen disease. Most schwannomas arise between the outer and inner layers of the MP.

Granular cell tumors mainly arise in the submucosa.

>   *Note*: Schwann cell hyperplasia and schwannomas are sometimes observed in the mucosa.

3.3 Gastrointestinal stromal tumors (GISTs)

The majority of GISTs are immunostain positive for KIT, but a few are immunostain negative for KIT and myogenic and neurogenic tumor markers. In addition, 80% of GISTs are immunostain positive for CD34. Differentiation between GISTs and myogenic tumors is sometimes difficult by H&E staining alone. GISTs may comprise spindle or epithelioid cells.

3.4 Lipoma and lipomatosis
3.5 Vascular tumor
3.6 Miscellaneous tumor

4 Lymphoma

Lymphoma is classified according to the WHO classification into B-cell lymphoma (MALT lymphoma, follicular lymphoma, mantle cell lymphoma, diffuse large B-cell lymphoma, Burkitt's lymphoma, others), T-cell lymphoma, and Hodgkin's lymphoma. For details, refer to the WHO classification: "Pathology and Genetics of Tumours of Haematopoietic and Lymphoid Tissues."

4.1 B-cell lymphoma
4.1.1 MALT lymphoma
4.1.2 Follicular lymphoma
4.1.3 Mantle cell lymphoma

4.1.4 Diffuse large B-cell lymphoma
4.1.5 Burkitt's lymphoma
4.1.6 Other lymphomas
4.2 T-cell lymphoma
4.3 Hodgkin lymphoma

5 Unclassifiable tumors

6 Metastatic tumors

7 Tumor-like lesions

7.1 Hyperplastic nodule

The macroscopic appearance of hyperplastic nodules is similar to that of hyperplastic polyps, but they lack luminal serration (Fig. 52).

7.2 Hyperplastic (metaplastic) polyp

Hyperplastic polyps and polyposis are characterized by elongation and dilatation of the tubules and luminal serration. Epithelial cells do not exhibit neoplastic atypia and contain abundant and faintly eosinophilic cytoplasm throughout the entire length of the tubules. High proliferative activity is observed in the lower half of the tubules (Fig. 53).

> Note: Non-neoplastic tubules may show misplacement to the submucosal layer.

7.3 Sessile serrated adenoma/polyp (SSA/P)

Sessile serrated adenoma/polyps are serrated lesions that cannot be clearly identified as tumors and contain 10% or more of the lesion area showing at least 2 of the following factors: 1) crypt dilation, 2) irregularly branching crypts, and 3) horizontally deformed basal area crypts (inverted "T-" and/or "L-" shaped crypts) (Fig. 54).

7.4 Juvenile polyp

Juvenile polyps comprise epithelial tubules, which may be dilated or cystic, and embedded in an excess of lamina propria. The superficial portion of the lamina propria is edematous and comprises proliferating and dilated capillaries, proliferating fibroblasts and fibrous tissue, and chronic inflammatory cell infiltrates. They may be complicated by hemorrhage or erosion (Fig. 55).

Juvenile polyps appear as reddish edematous elevations with necrotic tissue at the surface and may be sessile or pedunculated. They are observed in both children and adults.

> *Note*: A condition characterized by numerous juvenile polyps confined to the large intestine is called colorectal juvenile polyposis, and when juvenile polyps are also present in the stomach and small intestine, this condition is called gastrointestinal juvenile polyposis.

7.5 Inflammatory polyp and polyposis

Inflammatory polyps are non-neoplastic polyps that develop in association with inflammation and comprise pseudo- and regenerative polyps.

7.6 Inflammatory fibroid polyp

7.7 Inflammatory myoglandular polyp

7.8 Hamartomatous polyp

7.9 Mucosal prolapse syndrome

Mucosal prolapse syndrome is a condition characterized by capillary proliferation and dilatation and chronic inflammatory cell infiltrates, particularly in the superficial layer of the mucosa propria and fibromusculosis. Macroscopically, they are flat, elevated, ulcerative, or colitis cystica profunda types. The elevated type comprises dilated and proliferating glands and is usually accompanied by surface erosion and granulation tissue.

7.10 Cap polyposis

Macroscopic and histological features of cap polyposis are reminiscent of those of the elevated type of mucosal prolapse syndrome. However, cap polyposis is characterized by a wide range of localizations from the sigmoid colon to the rectum (occasionally extending to the right side of the colon), whereas mucosal prolapse syndrome is confined to the rectum.

7.11 Benign lymphoid polyp

Benign lymphoid polyps are polypoid lesions comprising circumscribed areas of hyperplasia of lymphoid follicles. The polyps are usually up to several millimeters in diameter. The most prevalent sites are the cecum and the rectum, and a condition in which multiple lesions are present is called polyposis. Multiple polyps are usually of a uniform size and less than 5 mm in diameter.

7.12 Endometriosis

7.13 Others

Heterotopic gastric mucosa, elastofibromatous polyp, colonic muco-submucosal elongated polyp, etc.

8 Hereditary tumors and gastrointestinal polyposis

8.1 Familial adenomatous polyposis

Familial adenomatous polyposis is an autosomal dominant disease in which *APC* mutations cause numerous colorectal adenomas and adenocarcinomas. Most cases develop countless small polyps, which develop into adenomas of the large intestine, duodenum, etc.

8.2 Lynch syndrome

Lynch syndrome was previously called hereditary non-polyposis colorectal cancer (HNPCC). It is a syndrome in which defects in the DNA mismatch repair gene cause colorectal cancer and endometrial carcinoma. The onset of colorectal cancer often occurs in young individuals and affects the right side of the colon.

8.3 Peutz-Jeghers syndrome

Peutz-Jeghers syndrome is a hereditary syndrome that is characterized by polyposis of the gastrointestinal tract and abnormal pigmentation of the skin and mucous membranes. Polyps develop in the stomach and the small and large intestines and comprise epithelial hyperplasia with various degrees of gland dilatation, accompanied by tree-like branching of the muscularis mucosae (Fig. 56).

They are non-neoplastic lesions.

> *Note*: Solitary polyps with histological features identical to those of the polyps in Peutz-Jeghers syndrome are called Peutz-Jeghers-type polyps.

8.4 Serrated polyposis/hyperplastic polyposis

Previously referred to as hyperplastic polyposis, serrated polyposis is characterized by small sessile lesions that are frequently 1 cm or less in size, and protruded tumors are rare. Large polyps often appear in the right side of the colon.

8.5 Cronkhite-Canada syndrome, Cronkhite-Canada polyp

Cronkhite-Canada syndrome is manifested by gastrointestinal polyposis, alopecia (generalized loss of hair), skin pigmentation, nail atrophy, and protein-losing gastroenteropathy. Multiple polyps are detected throughout the digestive tract, and the polyps comprise enlarged cystic glands containing eosinophilic material and edematous stroma (Fig. 57).

The mucosa between the polyps also contains edematous stroma and cystic glands.

8.6 Juvenile polyposis

8.7 Cowden syndrome: PTEN hamartoma syndrome (Cowden polyp)

Cowden syndrome is a hereditary disease characterized by multiple polyps throughout the digestive tract and is frequently accompanied by various benign skin lesions and carcinoma of the breast and thyroid gland.

The polyps in the large intestine are histologically similar to juvenile polyp.

B. Vermiform appendix

1 Benign epithelial tumor

Classified in accordance with tumors of the large intestine

2 Low-grade appendiceal mucinous neoplasm

Low-grade appendiceal mucinous neoplasms indicate tumors containing cells with abundant mucin production and a layer of columnar epithelial cells with low atypia (WHO classification, 2010). It is often difficult to determine the presence or absence of invasion and whether the tumor is benign or malignant (Fig. 58).

3 Malignant epithelial neoplasia

3.1 Adenocarcinoma: Classified in accordance with tumors of the large intestine

3.2 Goblet cell carcinoid

Cells resembling goblet cells proliferate in small aggregates or as individual cells. The onset is commonly in the vermiform appendix, and it often shows a concentric configuration in the appendiceal lumen. In this guideline, it is considered a subtype of adenocarcinoma (Fig. 59).

3.3 Carcinoid tumor, 4. Non-epithelial tumor, 5. Malignant lymphoma, 6. Tumor-like lesions are treated in accordance with the classification of colorectal tumors.

> *Note 1*: Several classifications have been proposed for appendiceal mucinous neoplasms; however, in the present classification, low-grade appendiceal mucinous neoplasms have been employed for consistency with the WHO classification. In the WHO classification, the disease concept of mucinous cystadenocarcinomas negates mucinous cystadenomas documented in the previous guidelines. Majority of mucinous cystadenomas and some mucinous cystadenocarcinomas are believed to correspond to low-grade appendiceal mucinous neoplasms. Adenocarcinomas with a high degree of atypia and marked mucin production are classified as mucinous carcinomas in accordance with the classification for colorectal tumors.
>
> *Note 2*: Tumors that produce mucin can cause pseudomyxoma peritonei.

C. Anal canal (including the perianal skin)

Macroscopically, the "surgical anal canal" is the region from the superior border of the puborectal slings to the anal verge. Histologically, this area extends from the superior border of the puborectal slings to the transitional part of the perirectal skin. The anal canal is separated into rectal, transitional, and squamous zones. In the squamous zone, the anal canal is devoid of cutaneous appendages and merges with the perianal skin. Anal glands are found from the submucosal layer to the sphincter muscle layer of the anal canal, with their openings into the anal sinuses (anal crypts).

1 Benign epithelial neoplasia

Adenomas and traditional serrated adenomas arising in the mucous membrane of the rectum are classified in accordance with adenomas of the large intestine. In the squamous zone, condyloma acuminatum (Fig. 60) and squamous cell papilloma occur. Tumors of cutaneous appendages, such as hidradenoma papilliferum, sometimes extend to the anal canal.

2 Squamous intraepithelial neoplasia

Lesions defined as squamous intraepithelial neoplasms are divided into low-grade intraepithelial neoplasia, high-grade intraepithelial neoplasia, and carcinoma in situ based on the structure of the squamous epithelium and cellular atypia. Alternatively, they are called "low-grade intraepithelial lesion (LSIL)" and "high-grade intraepithelial lesion (HSIL)," respectively. The condition where perianal squamous intraepithelial neoplasia is observed in the perianal skin is called Bowen's disease.

3 Malignant epithelial tumors
3.1 Adenocarcinoma
3.1.1 Rectal-type adenocarcinoma

Adenocarcinomas arising in the mucous membrane of the rectum are classified in accordance with those of the large intestine. In the event of mucinous carcinomas, differentiation with fistula cancer is required.

3.1.2 Extramural (perianal) adenocarcinoma

Adenocarcinomas associated with anorectal fistula develop in patients with a long history of anorectal fistula and are associated with Crohn's disease. These are often mucinous carcinomas; however, other histological types have also been reported (Fig. 61)

Adenocarcinomas of anal glands are rare tumors with a tubular structure and little mucin production

3.2 Squamous cell carcinoma

Squamous cell carcinomas arise between the transitional and squamous epithelium and are often associated with human papillomavirus (HPV). HPVs involved in the onset of squamous cell carcinoma of the anus, which is similar to cervical cancer, include high-risk HPV types, such as HPV16 and HPV18.

3.3 Adenosquamous carcinoma

Adenosquamous carcinomas contain components of both adenocarcinomas and squamous epithelium carcinomas and comprise carcinomas originating from the rectal mucosa and those originating between the transitional zone and squamous epithelium.

3.4 Carcinoid tumor

Classification is in accordance with that for colorectal tumors.

3.5 Endocrine cell carcinomas

Classification conforms to that for colorectal tumors, but there are also reports of endocrine cell carcinomas originating from squamous cell carcinomas.

3.6 Others

Verrucous, basal cell, and basaloid-squamous carcinomas have been reported.

4 Malignant melanoma

Malignant melanomas account for 1%–3% of malignancies of the anal canal and typically form elevated polypoid lesions; however, in advanced cases, ulcerative lesions are also observed. Tumor cell morphology can vary from epithelioid to fusiform cells. Lesions often produce melanin and are black; however, in some cases, melanin production is not noticeable (Fig. 62).

5 Extramammary Paget's disease

Extramammary Paget's disease lesions arise in apocrine-rich areas, such as the perianal skin and near the genitalia, and can extend to the anal canal. Tumor cells in nest formations or individual units are found at the base or spread through all layers of the squamous epithelium. These cells have large nuclei and abundant and clear cytoplasm (Fig. 63). Extramammary Paget's disease may require differentiation from rectal cancer showing pagetoid progression in the perianal skin.

6 Non-epithelial tumor: Mesenchymal tumor
Classified in accordance with tumors of the large intestine

7 Malignant lymphoma
Classified in accordance with tumors of the large intestine

8 Tumor-like lesion
Tumor-like lesions are classified in accordance with tumors of the large intestine and include internal hemorrhoids, retention cysts, and fibroepithelial polyps.

9 Others

2 Histological assessment of biopsy specimens (Group classification)

The classification applies only to colorectal biopsy specimens, including hot biopsy specimens, that have been endoscopically obtained and not to polypectomy, mucosal resection, or surgical specimens. It also applies only to epithelial lesions. This Group classification is intended to clarify the diagnostic (disease) category of lesions, and, in principle, when the diagnosis is made using biopsy, the diagnostic term is recorded and the Group classification is recorded along with it.

Group details
- Group X: Inadequate material for histological diagnosis
    No epithelial component is included in the biopsy specimen or the specimen is inadequate as a result of being severely damaged by the biopsy procedure.
- Group 1: Normal mucosa and inflamed or hyperplastic mucosa
- Group 2: Lesions in which it is difficult to determine whether the lesion is tumorous (adenoma, adenocarcinoma) or non-tumorous based on cell atypia, structural atypia, etc., are included in this group. Atypical gland ducts that appear in association with mucosal prolapse syndrome, etc., correspond to such lesions.
- Group 3: A range of lesions in terms of cellular or structural atypia is included in this group, and lesions that have been judged to be benign neoplasia belong to this group.
- Group 4: (1) A sufficient amount of tumor tissue is biopsied but a definite diagnosis of carcinoma cannot be made on the basis of architectural and cytological atypia.
    (2) Carcinoma is suspected but the biopsy specimen is too small to make a definite diagnosis.

(3) Carcinoma is suspected but the biopsy specimen is too severely damaged to make a definite diagnosis.

Group 5: The lesion is definitely diagnosed as carcinoma based on its nuclear atypia (enlarged, irregularly contoured, hyperchromatic nuclei, loss of nuclear polarity, large nucleoli), cytoplasmic abnormalities (marked mucin depletion, basophilic cytoplasm), and abnormal duct structure (irregular branching, tortuosity, fusion, etc.).

Note 1: When group classification is difficult because of reasons such as the amount of tissue that has been collected is small, it is important not to force a classification but to record only the tissue findings (tissue diagnosis) and inform the clinician of the need for a repeat biopsy, etc.

Note 2: Sometimes, atypical epithelium appears against a background of chronic inflammation in ulcerative colitis or another inflammatory bowel disease (IBD) in which it is difficult to differentiate between tumorous and non-tumorous, but when the presence of IBD is clinically and pathologically clear, it is preferable to record the class of degree of atypia according to the Histopathological Evaluation Criteria for the Atypical Epithelium that Occurs in Ulcerative Colitis* and not to use the Group classification. Nevertheless, even when this type of atypical epithelium is present, when the presence of IBD is unclear at the time of biopsy, the diagnosis is sometimes made using the Group classification (particularly Group 2). In such instances, the class of degree of atypia can by recorded later at the stage when a definite diagnosis of IBD has been made. In addition, ordinary adenomas and carcinomas sometimes also develop in patients with IBD, and when they do, the Group classification is used.

*Ministry of Health and Welfare Special-Disease Intractable Inflammatory Bowel Disorder Survey Study Group: Histopathological Evaluation Criteria for the Atypical Epithelium that Occurs in Ulcerative Colitis: Proposal for New Evaluation Criteria Designed for Application to Surveillance Colonoscopy. J Jpn Soc Colo-proctol, 47: 547-551, 1994.

Note 3: Because Group 2 includes tissue in which it is difficult to differentiate between tumorous and non-tumorous tissues, the need to collect detailed clinical information or to perform a repeat biopsy should be considered.

Ref: Vienna classification of gastrointestinal epithelial neoplasia

The Vienna classification applies to the diagnosis of both biopsy and resected specimens. Epithelial neoplastic lesions associated with IBD can also be classified by this classification.

Category 1	Negative for neoplasia/dysplasia
Category 2	Indefinite for neoplasia/dysplasia
Category 3	Non-invasive low-grade neoplasia (low grade adenoma/dysplasia)
Category 4	Non-invasive high-grade neoplasia
	4.1 High-grade adenoma/dysplasia
	4.2 Non-invasive carcinoma (carcinoma in situ) *
	4.3 Suspicion of invasive carcinoma
Category 5	Invasive neoplasia (carcinoma)
	5.1 Intramucosal carcinoma **
	5.2 Submucosal carcinoma or beyond

* Non-invasive indicates no distinct evidence of invasion
** Neoplasia which shows invasion to the lamina propria or muscularis mucosae
According to the WHO classification, "non-invasive neoplasia" is termed as "intraepithelial neoplasia (dysplasia)."
(cited from Schlemper RJ, et al. The Vienna classification of gastrointestinal epithelial neoplasia. Gut 47: 251-255, 2000.)

3 Handling of resected specimens

3.1 Handling of biopsy materials

After a biopsy is taken, the specimen must be promptly immersed in 10% neutral buffered formalin solution. The recommended fixing time is a minimum of 6 h and a maximum of 72 h.

3.2 Macroscopic examination and handling of surgically resected specimens

(1) Macroscopic inspections and palpation of the serosal surface
  - Evaluation of presence or absence of serosal or mesenteric invasions and lymph node metastasis.
  - In cases of invasion and/or metastasis being present, determine the sites, the distance from the edge of the lesion to the bilateral cutting edge of the resected specimen, the spread of the invasion or metastasis, and its properties.
  - Take as many lymph nodes out from the resected specimen as possible and immerse them in 10% neutral buffered formalin solution, separating by each lymph node station.

(2) Incision of the resected specimen
  - Resected specimen of the rectum should be cut longitudinally at the anterior side.
  - Resected specimen of the colon should be also cut longitudinally at the antimesenteric side.
  - If the tumor lays on the above mentioned cutline, change the line to avoid cutting into the lesion.

(3) Extension of the incised specimen.

With the mucosa facing up, extend it to approximately the same length as that in the living body on a securing plate and then affix using rustproof pins. Make sketches and take unmagnified photographs with a ruler in place.

(4) Measuring tumors and resected specimen (Fig. 19)

  (a) Distance to the cut end
   - Distances between the tumor edge and both proximal and distal cut ends are measured.
   - For rectal specimens, the distance from the lower edge of the tumor to the dentate line and to the edge of the cut skin is measured.

  (b) Size and height
    Maximum diameter × diameter orthogonal to the maximum diameter × height (mm)

  (c) Tumor intestinal annular proportion
    (Maximum transverse diameter of the tumor/intestinal transverse diameter) × 100 (%)

  (d) Macroscopic tumor types
   - When ulcers or tumor parts in the mucosa are merged, their sizes should be noted.
   - For 0-I types, the shape of the head, size, presence of a stalk, and length should also be noted.

(5) Fixing specimens

Fix each specimen with fresh 10% neutral buffered formalin solution; ideally, fixing should occur within 3 hours of specimen collection. If there is a delay before fixing, then the sample should be temporarily stored in a refrigerator within 30 minutes of sampling, along with protection from drying. The recommended fixing time is a minimum of 6 hours and a maximum of 72 hours.

(6) Processing fixed specimens

  (a) Macroscopic observations and photographs

    Macroscopically observe, measure, record, and photograph the specimens alongside a ruler in the same manner as done for fresh specimen.

  (b) Cutting (Fig. 20)
   - The lesions are cut into sections to obtain tissues that were thought to be necessary for procuring histological images of the deepest part of the cancer invasion and the mucosal surface.
   - As a rule, cut tumors at approximately 5–6 mm intervals along the long axis of the intestine.
   - Depending on the situation, it is also acceptable to section the tumor at right angles to its long axis or along its maximum diameter.
   - Prior to selecting a tissue slice for sampling, examine the cut surface and determine the

depth of invasion and presence of invasions in the serosa, adventitia, mesentery, and adjacent organs and whether lymph nodes are adhering to the intestinal tract. Measure and record the distance from the cut surface to the proximal and distal cut ends and from the detached surface to the tumor.
· In parallel, completely resect small lesions and lesions judged to be early cancers with a width of 2–4 mm and use the whole tumor as the tissue sample.
· After reconstructing the sectioned blocks (specimens), it is recommended that photos be retaken from the mucosal side.
· Partition the appendix either longitudinally (along the long axis of the appendix) or transversely (cross-sectional slices) depending on the lesion type. Making cross-sectional slices to the appendix renders the relationship to the mesentery easier to view.
· As a rule, when taking photos or drawing sketches, orient these so that the mucosal surface is on the top and the distal (anal) portions are on the left.

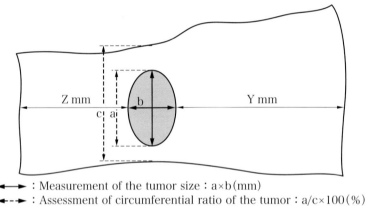

⟶ : Measurement of the tumor size : a×b (mm)
⟵--⟶ : Assessment of circumferential ratio of the tumor : a/c×100(%)

Fig. 19 Measurement of the resected specimen

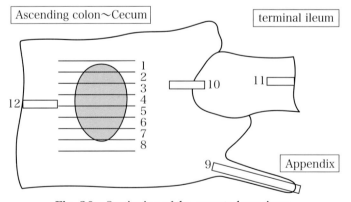

Fig. 20 Sectioning of the resected specimen

・During histopathological examinations, after photographing partition lines, map the extent of tumor development and extent of invasion and record the tumor size (the longest diameter and the shortest diameter orthogonal to the longest diameter).

3.3 Handling of endoscopically resected specimens

Endoscopic resection is classified into 2 categories as follows: En block resection is defined as one piece removal of entire lesion, and piecemeal resection is defined as multiple pieces removal.

(1) Extending and fixing specimens
  (a) Superficial-type lesions

    After resecting and clearly noting the proximal and distal sides, promptly extend and fix the sample in accordance with the diameter observed by endoscopy findings and immerse in 10% neutral buffered formalin. The recommended fixing time is a minimum of 6 hours and a maximum of 72 hours.

  (b) Protruded-type lesions (polyps)

    Immerse in 10% neutral buffered formalin as is. The recommended fixing time is a minimum of 6 hours and a maximum of 72 hours.

(2) Processing fixed specimens
  (a) Macroscopic observations and records

    Record the size of the endoscopic resection specimen (longest and shortest axis), tumor size (long diameter and the short diameter orthogonal to the long diameter), type according to macroscopic observation, presence or absence of stalks and their lengths, mucosal pattern and color tone, and the distance from the resection margin to the lesion. It is acceptable to dye the cut edge to evaluate the margin.

  (b) Excisions (Fig. 21)

    Pedunculated lesions with a stalk width of 2 mm or greater
- In consideration of the coarse-cut paraffin blocks, cut 1 mm from the center of the stalk at 2 mm intervals.
- All tissue fragments other than the central part should be used to prepare pathological specimens.

    Pedunculated lesions with a stalk width of less than 2 mm
- Do not cut the stalk, but embed the whole stalk in a paraffin block, and use coarse and fine cuts to reveal the center of the stalk.

    Sessile protrusion- and superficial type lesions
- Resected specimens are cut into sections to obtain tissues for pathological evaluation of the portion closest to the horizontal margin, and then, completely resect at 2–3

mm intervals parallel to the partition.
- When excising parts macroscopically suspected of being submucosal invasions, cut approximately 1 mm of the portion presumed to be the deepest invasion.

(c) Photography and mapping
- For reconstruction, take unmagnified photographs with a ruler before and after the excision.
- During histopathological examinations, after photographing with partition lines, map the extent of tumor development and invasion and record the tumor size (the longest diameter and the shortest diameter orthogonal to the longest diameter).

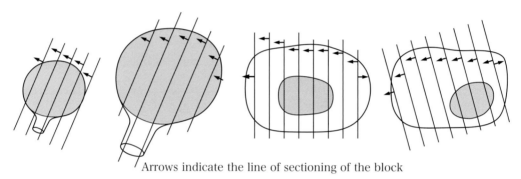

Arrows indicate the line of sectioning of the block

Fig. 21 Sectioning of a endoscopically resected specimen

Supplementary histology atlas

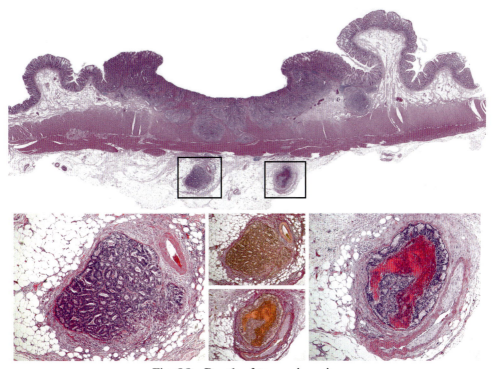

Fig. 22 Depth of tumor invasion

Moderately differentiated tubular adenocarcinoma infiltrating to the muscular propria; however, two discontinuous cancer cell nests (EX) can be seen in the subserosa (Top). These cancer cell nests are surrounded by elastic fibers on high magnification and staining with elastica van Gieson. Those cancer nests are venous invasion that located deeper than direct invasion (Bottom). In such cases of direct cancer invasion to the musclaris propria with venous invasion in the submucosa, the depth of invasion is judged as pT3, where EX exists, and recorded as pT3 (V)-MP.

82   III. Explanation of pathological items [Supplement: Histology Atlas]

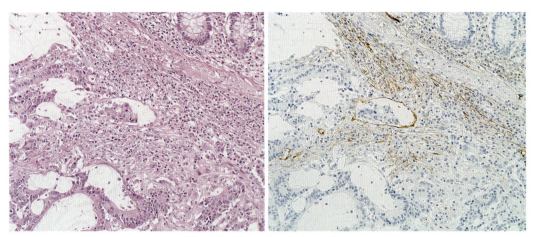

Fig. 23 Lymphatic invasion

Tumor cell invasion can be seen in the lumen lined by lymphatic endothelium. Intraluminal endothelium cells are D2-40-positive. D2-40 expression can be found in the surrounding stromal fibroblasts; therefore, it is important to verify the expression in endothelial cells.
Left: HE staining, Right: D2-40 immunostaining

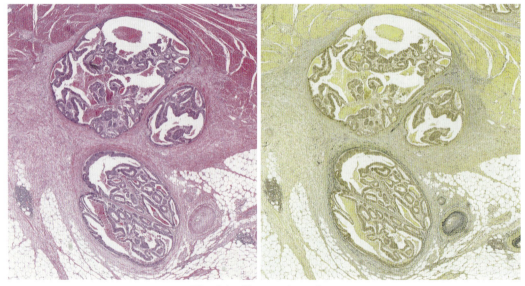

Fig. 24 Venous invasion

Cancer cell nests can be seen surrounded by a vascular-like structure located near the existing arteries. Elastica van Gieson (EVG) staining confirms lamina elastica covering half or more of the circumference, and the lesion is defined as "V."
Left: HE staining, Right: EVG staining

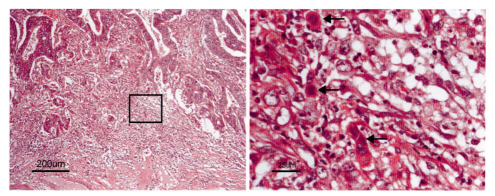

Fig. 25 Tumor budding

Budding (arrow on the Right). A cancer cell nest consisting of one or fewer than five cells that has infiltrated the interstitium at the invasive margin of the cancer is seen. The Right is the square area on the Left.

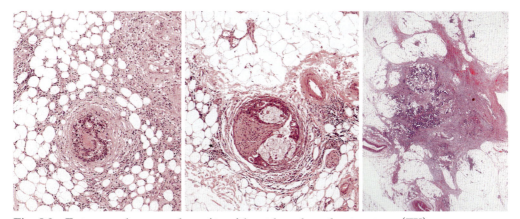

Fig. 26 Extramural cancer deposits without lymph node structure (EX)

Left: Vascular invasion lesion; Middle: Perineural invasion lesion, Right: EX other than vascular/perineural invasion lesions (tumor nodule: ND)

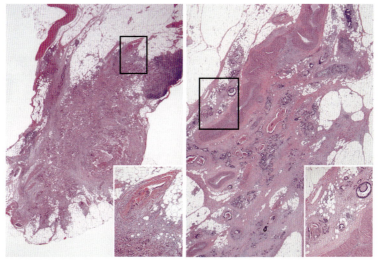

Fig. 27 ND accompanied with venous/perineural invasion
Left: ND(V+), Right: ND(Pn+)

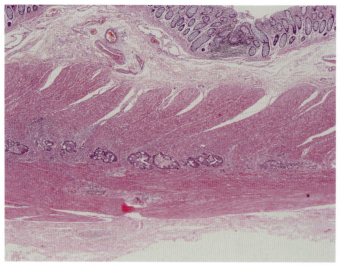

Fig. 28 Perineural invasion (Pn)
Intramural Pn. Histological finding of cancer nests spreading along with replacing the Auerbach nerve plexus.

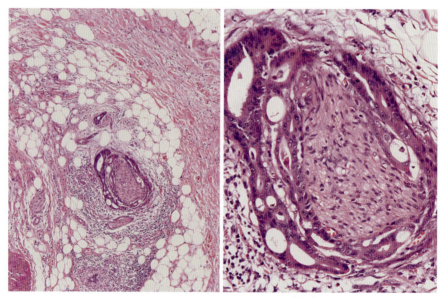

Fig. 29 Perineural invasion (Pn)
Extramural Pn forming a solitary lesion.

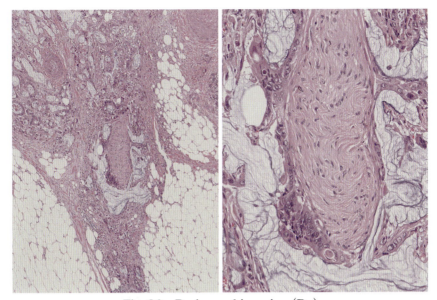

Fig. 30 Perineural invasion (Pn)
Extramural Pn observed in the body of the primary lesion.

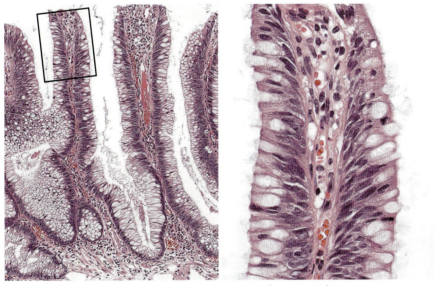

Fig. 31 Tubular adenoma (low grade)
Low-grade tubular adenoma with abundant mucin production. High proliferation activity is seen in the upper portion of the glands, and neoplastic cells are differentiating into mucin-producing cells at the bottom (Left). Pseudostratification of spindle-shaped nuclei is seen in the area of high proliferative activity, but their polarity is maintained (Right).

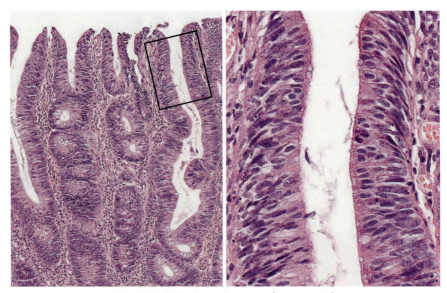

Fig. 32 Tubular adenoma (low grade)

Low-grade tubular adenoma with scanty mucin production. High proliferative activity is seen in the upper portion of the glands (Left). Spindle-shaped nuclei in the area of high proliferative activity are pseudostratified (Right), but in the lower portion, these are regularly arranged in the basal half of the gland lumen (Left).

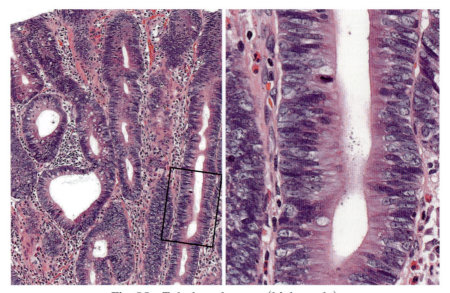

Fig. 33 Tubular adenoma (high grade)

High-grade tubular adenoma with low mucin production. The gland duct appears expanded and tortuous. Intense proliferation is observed in the surface layer, where pseudostratified nuclei are noticeable with much mitosis (Left). Even the regions with low proliferation activity show mitosis occasionally (Right). The extent of nuclear pseudostratification is approximately half of the thickness of the epithelium, and nuclei are ovoid (increase in the short nucleic axis) and contain light and small basophilic nucleoli.

Supplementary histology atlas 87

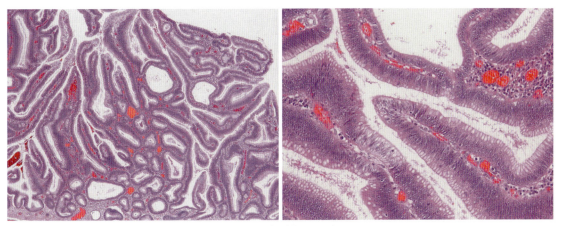

Fig. 34 Tubulovillous adenoma

Tubular structure showing dilation and tortuosity, intermixed with a pointed villous structure. From the middle layer to the surface, an area can be seen with high proliferative activity, where nuclei exhibit pseudostratification (Left). Spindle-shaped nuclei are orderly arranged with polarity maintained in approximately half of the basal side (Right).

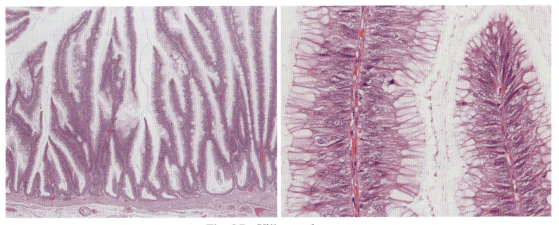

Fig. 35 Villous adenoma

The epithelium has a pointed villous (papillary) structure with a narrow lamina propria and a base adjacent to the muscularis mucosa (Left). Each individual villous structure has a vascular axis with poor stromal components. Nuclei are irregularly arranged in approximately half of the basal side with small nucleoli (Right).

88 III. Explanation of pathological items [Supplement: Histology Atlas]

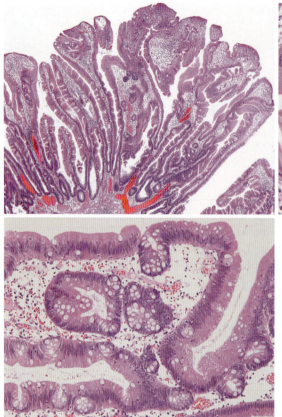

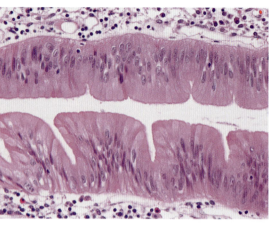

Fig. 36 Serrated adenoma
A polyp showing papillary growth entirely. A luminal serrated structure can be seen at low power magnification (Upper Left). Tumor cells comprise eosinophilic and mildly eosinophilic cells with short Spindle-shaped nuclei and few goblet cells. In the serrated area, nuclei are isolated from the basal side and show pseudostratification (Upper Right). Ectopic crypt formation is considered another characteristic finding (Bottom).

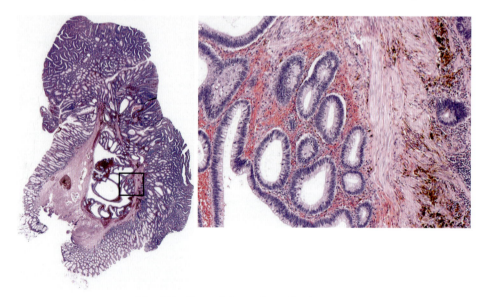

Fig. 37 Pseudoinvasion of adenoma
Tubular adenoma glands with low-grade atypia showing pseudoinvasion to the submucosa (Left). A layer of the lamina propria is present in the atypical gland area with pseudoinvasion. Bleeding and hemosiderin deposition can be seen in the interstitium (Right).

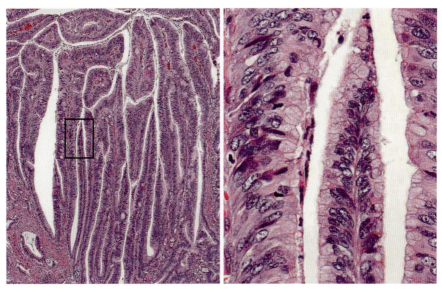

Fig. 38 Papillary adenocarcinoma (pap)
Advanced cancer showing a papillary or villous pattern of growth (Left). Enlarged round or oval nuclei (enlarged nuclear short axis) with pseudostratification are seen. Mucous vacuoles are seen at the luminal side of the cytoplasm (Right).

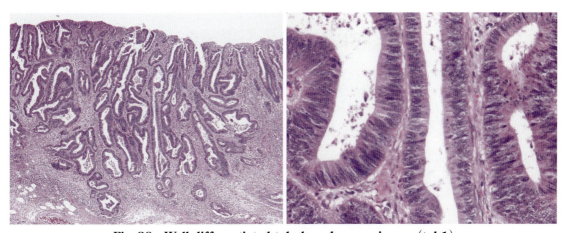

Fig. 39 Well differentiated tubular adenocarcinoma (tub1)
Invasive growth of adenocarcinoma primarily comprising cells with a clear tubular structure (Left). Nuclear polarity is relatively maintained; however, the nuclei have enlarged fusiform to oval shape, crude chromatin, and several prominent nucleoli (Right).

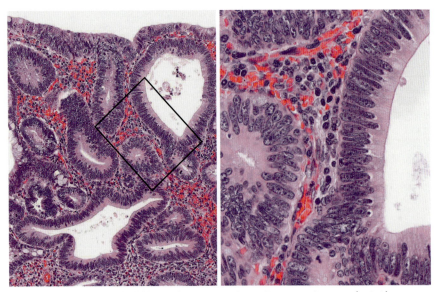

Fig. 40 Well differentiated tubular adenocarcinoma (tub1)
Cancerous tubules are dilated and tortuous (Left). Nuclear pseudostratification slightly exceeds half the height of the epithelium. Cancer cells have enlarged hyperchromatic nuclei with prominent nucleoli. The cytoplasm is eosinophilic with scanty mucin production.

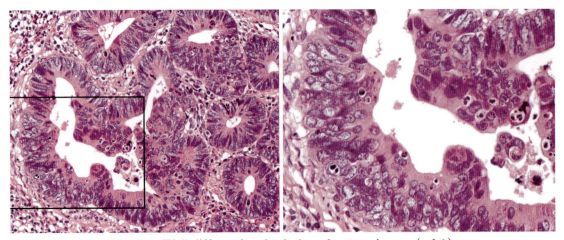

Fig. 41 Well differentiated tubular adenocarcinoma (tub1)
Well differentiated tubular adenocarcinoma with high-grade cellular atypia and scarce mucin production. Round or oval nuclei show severe pseudostratification.

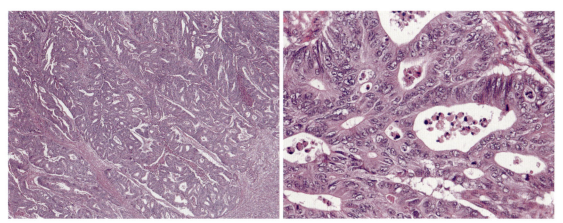

Fig. 42　Moderately differentiated tubular adenocarcinoma (tub2)
Moderately differentiated adenocarcinoma proliferating with various-sized cribriform patterns (Left). The tumor comprises columnar cells with enlarged nuclei and prominent nucleoli, and necrotic cells are retained in the ductal lumen (Right).

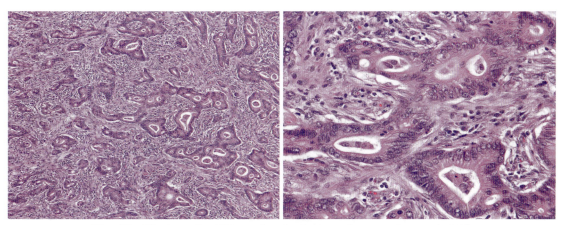

Fig. 43　Moderately differentiated tubular adenocarcinoma (tub2)
Moderately differentiated adenocarcinoma proliferating with moderate to small tubular structures. Severe fibrosis can be seen in the background (Left). Ducts comprising columnar cells with small round nucrei are irregularly anastomosing (Right).

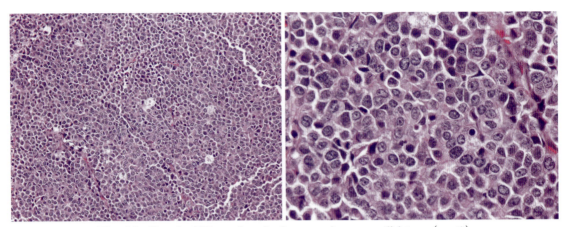

Fig. 44 **Poorly differentiated adenocarcinoma: solid type (por1)**

Tumor with cancer cells showing solid growth and little stroma (Left). Nuclei are round or oval, with mildly eosinophilic and partially foamy cytoplasm.

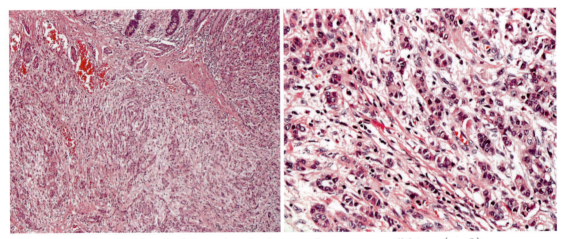

Fig. 45 **Poorly differentiated adenocarcinoma: non-solid type (por2)**

Cancer cells form a predominantly trabecular structure and show less tubule formation and are rich in fibrous stroma (por2). Hardly any mucin production is seen.

Supplementary histology atlas 93

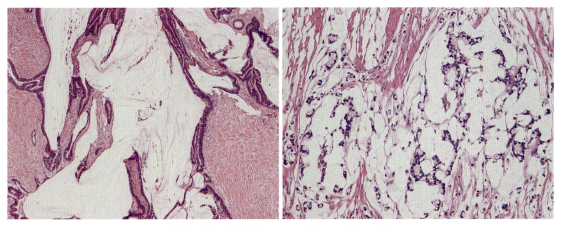

Fig. 46 Mucinous carcinoma（muc）

Tumor-forming mucous nodules (mucous lake). Mucinous carcinoma is divided into well differentiated mucinous carcinoma, including tubular and papillary adenocarcinoma (Left), and poorly differentiated mucinous carcinoma, comprising poorly differentiated tubular adenocarcinoma and/or signet-ring cell carcinoma with abundant extracellular mucous secretion (Right).

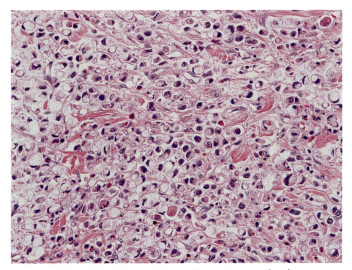

Fig. 47 Signet-ring cell carcinoma（sig）

Cancer cells containing abundant intracellular mucous and poor extracellular secretion.

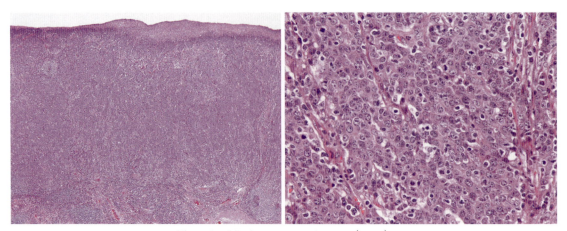

Fig. 48   Medullary carcinoma (med)
Poorly differentiated adenocarcinoma with solid, sheet-like proliferation surrounded by severe lymphocyte infiltration (Left). Cells with eosinophilic cytoplasm and nuclei with prominent nucleoli and conspicuous intraepithelial lymphocyte invasion (Right). It was classified as poorly differentiated adenocarcinoma, solid type (por1) in the 7th Japanese edition and 2nd English edition of JCCRC.

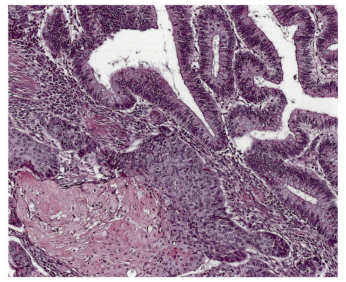

Fig. 49   Adenosquamous carcinoma (asc)
Both Well differentiated tubular adenocarcinoma and squamous carcinoma can be seen.

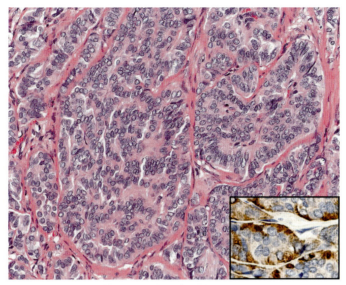

Fig. 50　Carcinoid tumor

Carcinoid tumor of the rectum (shows submucosal component) comprising uniform small cells with round or oval nuclei forming ribbon-like and trabecular structures with a highly vascular stroma. In general, mitotic figures are infrequent. The tumor contains numerous chromogranin A-positive cells (Inset).

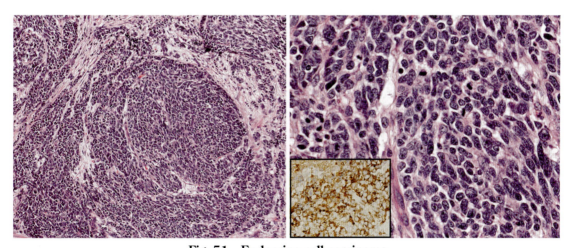

Fig. 51　Endocrine cell carcinoma

The tumor comprises rather uniform small- or medium sized cancer cells containing scanty cytoplasm that have formed a sheet-like or large solid structure and contains a highly vascular stroma (Right and Left). In general, cancer cell nuclei are larger and more hyperchromatic than carcinoid tumor nuclei. Although the nucleoli are not conspicuous, there are numerous mitotic figures. Several chromogranin-positive cells can be seen (Inset).

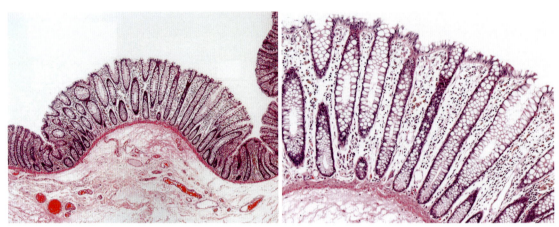

Fig. 52　Hyperplastic nodule
A localized area comprising hyperplastic glands without luminal serration is seen.

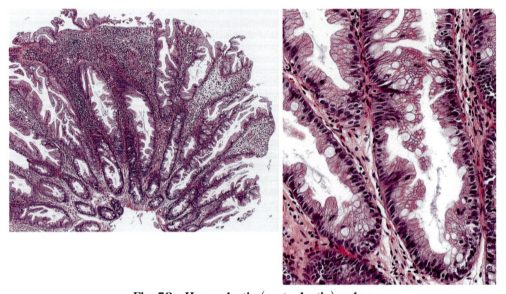

Fig. 53　Hyperplastic (metaplastic) polyp
Elevated lesion exhibits luminal serration. The epithelial cells do not exhibit neoplastic atypia and contain faintly eosinophilic cytoplasm. High proliferative activity is seen in the lower portion of the tubules.

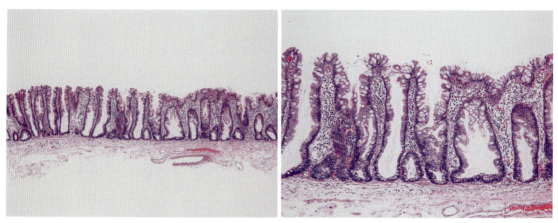

Fig. 54　Sessile serrated adenoma/polyp (SSA/P)

A serrated lesion resembling a hyperplastic polyp; however, crypt dilation, irregular branching, and horizontally deformed basal area crypts (inverted "T-" or "L-" shaped crypts) can be seen.

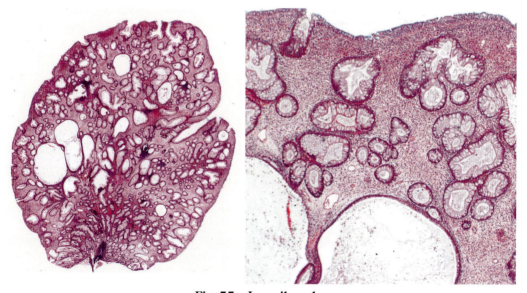

Fig. 55　Juvenile polyp

The polyp comprises a large amount of stroma and dilated tubules (Left). The superficial lamina propria is expanded by proliferation and dilatation of capillaries, fibroblast, and fibrous tissue and contains rich stromal cells as a result of chronic inflammatory cell infiltrates. Mild cystic dilatation of the tubules is seen. The interposition of muscularis mucosae is not observed.

98   III. Explanation of pathological items [Supplement: Histology Atlas]

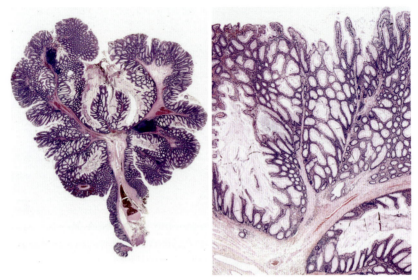

Fig. 56   Peutz-Jeghers syndrome
The polyp comprises hyperplastic epithelial cells with dilated tubules accompanied by tree-like branching of the muscularis mucosa.

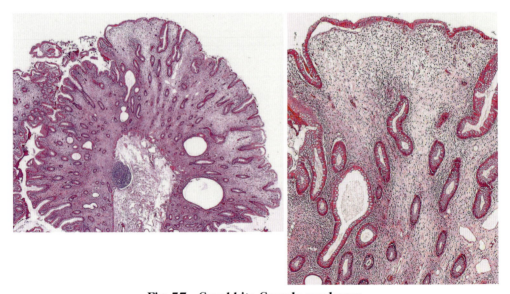

Fig. 57   Cronkhite-Canada syndrome
The lamina propria is highly edematous and contains mild to moderate chronic inflammatory infiltrates. Elongation and dilatation of glands are also seen, causing diffuse marked thickening of the mucosa. The thickening is the most severe at the top of the semilunar folds and usually appears as a polypoid lesion.

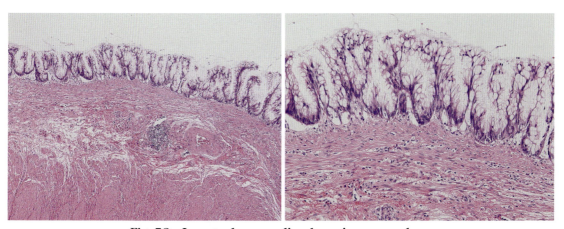

Fig. 58　Low-grade appendiceal mucinous neoplasm

Low papillary growth of a layer of mucous-producing cells (Left). Mild cellular atypia can be seen (Right).

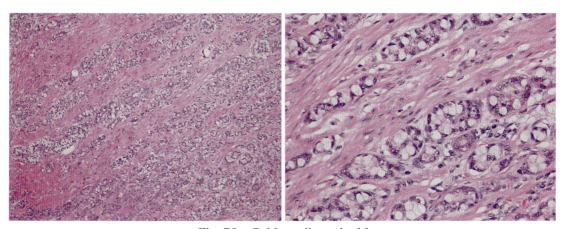

Fig. 59　Goblet cell carcinoid

Mucous-producing cells resembling goblet cells proliferate as small clusters or trabecular cells. While the name "carcinoid" remains, it is considered as a subtype of adenocarcinoma.

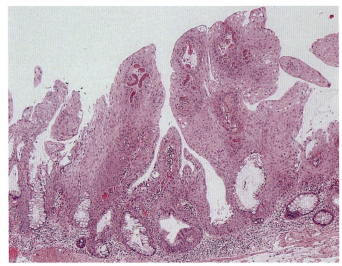

Fig. 60 Condyloma acuminatum of the anal canal
Papillary proliferation of squamous epithelial cells can be seen, with clearly differentiated surface and little cellular atypia.

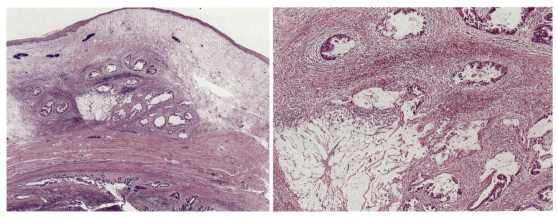

Fig. 61 Adenocarcinoma associated with anal fistula
Proliferation of adenocarcinoma can be seen extending from below the squamous epithelium to within the internal sphincter and deeper along the anal fistula (Left). This is a well differentiated adenocarcinoma with mucinous carcinoma components (Right).

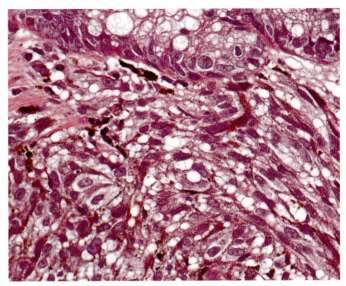

Fig. 62 Malignant melanoma

Melanin pigments are present in the tumor cells. The nuclei are oval or spindle-shaped and contain distinct nucleoli.

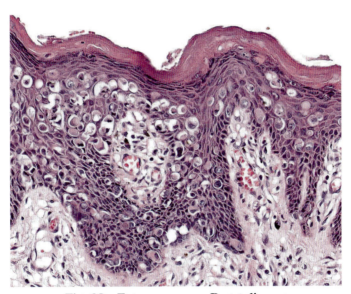

Fig. 63 Extramammary Paget disease

Numerous Paget cells (round to oval cells with abundant faintly eosinophilic cytoplasm and enlarged nuclei) are seen in the epidermis.

Supplements

- **TNM Classification of malignant tumours**
  Carcinoma of the colon and rectum
  Carcinoma of the appendix
  Carcinoma of the anal canal
  Well-differentiated neuroendocrine tumours (G1 and G2)
    of the colon and rectum, and the appendix
- **Summary of findings**
- **Checklist for pathological report**
- **List of abbreviations**

Supplement 1 TNM Classification of malignant tumours
Eighth Edition, 2017, Wiley-Blackwell, Chichester UK

Supplement 1-1 Carcinoma of the colon and rectum (ICD-O-3 C18-C20)

T Primary Tumour

TX   Primary tumour cannot be assessed

T0   No evidence of primary tumour

Tis Carcinoma in situ: invasion of lamina propria

T1   Tumour invades submucosa

T2   Tumour invades muscularis propria

T3   Tumour invades subserosa or into non-peritonealized pericolic or perirectal tissues

T4   Tumour directly invades other organs or structures and/or perforates visceral peritoneum

  T4a   Tumour perforates visceral peritoneum

  T4b   Tumour directly invades other organs or structures

N Regional Lymph Nodes

NX   Regional lymph nodes cannot be assessed

N0   No regional lymph node metastasis

N1   Metastasis in 1 to 3 regional lymph nodes

  N1a   Metastasis in 1 regional lymph node

  N1b   Metastasis in 2 to 3 regional lymph nodes

  N1c   Tumour deposit(s), i.e., satellites, in the subserosa, or in non-peritonealized pericolic or perirectal soft tissue without regional lymph node metastasis

N2   Metastasis in 4 or more regional lymph nodes

  N2a   Metastasis in 4-6 regional lymph nodes

  N2b   Metastasis in 7 or more regional lymph nodes

M Distant Metastasis

M0   No distant metastasis

M1   Distant metastasis

  M1a   Metastasis confined to one organ (e.g., liver, lung, ovary, non-regional lymph node(s)) without peritoneal metastases

  M1b   Metastasis in more than one organ

  M1c   Metastasis to the peritoneum with or without other organ involvement

Stage

Stage	T	N	M
Stage 0	Tis	N0	M0
Stage I	T1, T2	N0	M0
Stage II	T3, T4	N0	M0
Stage IIA	T3	N0	M0
Stage IIB	T4a	N0	M0
Stage IIC	T4b	N0	M0
Stage III	Any T	N1, N2	M0
Stage IIIA	T1, T2	N1	M0
	T1	N2a	M0
Stage IIIB	T1, T2	N2b	M0
	T2, T3	N2a	M0
	T3, T4a	N1	M0
Stage IIIC	T3, T4a	N2b	M0
	T4a	N2a	M0
	T4b	N1, N2	M0
Stage IV	Any T	Any N	M1
Stage IVA	Any T	Any N	M1a
Stage IVB	Any T	Any N	M1b
Stage IVC	Any T	Any N	M1c

Stage of carcinoma of the colon and rectum

M-Distant metastasis			M0				M1		
							M1a	M1b	M1c
N-Regional lymph nodes		N0	N1 (N1a/N1b/N1c)	N2a	N2b		Any N		
T-Primary tumour category	Tis	0							
	T1	I	IIIA				IVA	IVB	IVC
	T2			IIIB					
	T3	IIA							
	T4a	IIB			IIIC				
	T4b	IIC							

Source: TNM Classification of Malignant Tumours. Eighth Edition, 2017, Wiley-Blackwell, Chichester UK.

Comparison between JCCRC and the TNM classification

	JCCRC	TNM classification*
Depth of tumor invasion	TX: Depth of tumor invasion cannot be assessed T0: No evidence of primary tumor Tis: Tumor is confined to the mucosa and does not invade the submucosa T1a: Tumor is confined to the submucosa (SM), and invasion is within 1000 μm T1b: Tumor is confined to the submucosa (SM), and invasion is 1000 μm or more, but it does not extend to the muscularis propria (MP) T2: Tumor invasion to, but not beyond, MP T3: Tumor invades beyond the MP. In sites with the serosa, the tumor invades the subserosa (SS) In sites with no serosa, the tumor invades the adventitia (A). T4: Tumor invades or perforates the serosa (SE) or has directly invaded other organs or structures (SI/AI) T4a: Tumor invades or perforates the serosa (SE) T4b: Tumor directly invades adjacent organs	TX: Primary tumour cannot be assessed T0: No evidence of primary tumour Tis: Carcinoma in situ: invasion of lamina propria T1: Tumour invades submucosa T2: Tumour invades muscularis propria T3: Tumour invades subserosa or into non-peritonealized pericolic or perirectal tissues T4a: Tumour perforates visceral peritoneum T4b: Tumour directly invades other organs or structures
	Note: Of EX, vascular/perineural invasion lesions are used to determine the depth of invasion.	*Note*: Tumour deposits are not used to determine the depth of invasion.

Lymph node metastasis	NX: Lymph node metastasis cannot be assessed
	N0: No regional lymph node metastasis
	N1: 3 or fewer metastases in pericolic/perirectal and intermediate lymph nodes
	   N1a: Metastasis in 1 lymph node
	   N1b: Metastasis in 2-3 lymph nodes
	
	N2: 4 or more metastases in pericolic/perirectal and intermediate lymph nodes
	   N2a: Metastasis in 4-6 lymph nodes
	   N2b: Metastasis in 7 or more lymph nodes
	
	N3: Metastasis in the main lymph nodes observed. In cancer of the lower rectum, metastasis in the main and/or lateral lymph nodes is observed
		NX: Regional lymph nodes cannot be assessed
		N0: No regional lymph node metastasis
		N1: Metastasis in 1 to 3 regional lymph nodes
		   N1a: Metastasis in 1 regional lymph node
		   N1b: Metastasis in 2 to 3 regional lymph nodes
		   N1c: Tumour deposit (s), i.e., satellites, in the subserosa, or in non-peritonealized pericolic or perirectal soft tissue without regional lymph node metastasis
		N2: Metastasis in 4 or more regional lymph nodes
		   N2a: Metastasis in 4-6 regional lymph nodes
		   N2b: Metastasis in 7 or more regional lymph nodes

	Note: Of EX, tumor nodules (ND) are treated as lymph nodes, and the number of ND is added to the number of lymph node metastases.	*Note*: Of tumour deposits, only those in which the lymph nodes were considered by the pathologists to be totally replaced by cancer are treated as lymph nodes, and their number is added to the number of lymph node metastases.

	JCCRC	TNM classification*

Distant metastasis	M0: No distant metastasis observed.
	M1: Distant metastasis observed
	    M1a: Distant metastasis confined in one organ. Peritoneal metastasis not present.
	    M1b: Distant metastasis in more than one organ. Peritoneal metastasis not present.
	    M1c: Presence of peritoneal metmetastasis.
	        M1c1: Metastasis to the peritoneum only.
	        M1c2: Metastasis to the peritoneum with other distant metastasis.
		M0: No distant metastasis
		M1: Distant metastasis
		    M1a: Metastasis confined to one organ (e.g., liver, lung, ovary, non-regional node(s)) without peritoneal metastases
		    M1b: Metastasis in more than one organ
		    M1c: Metastasis to the peritoneum with or without other organ involvement

	EX includes localized lesions comprising lymphatic invasion, venous invasion, perineural invasion (vascular/perineural invasion lesions), and other lesions (tumor nodule: ND).(Page 37). When judging depth of tumor invasion, the TNM classifications are different from the JCCRC, and the TNM classification do not consider vascular invasion. For example, pathological T factor of tumors that directly invade to SM with venous invasion in MP is pT2. But this is pT1 as per the TNM classification, which does not consider venous invasion. Information on depth of tumor invasion and vascular invasion in such cases are described as follows. JCCRC: pT2 (V)-SM (Page 12-13) TNM classification: pT1, V1 (muscularis propria) Furthermore, perineural invasion are measured as depth of tumor invasion by TNM classifications as well as the JCCRC.	Tumour deposits (satellites) are discrete macroscopic or microscopic nodules of cancer in the pericolorectal adipose tissue's lymph drainage area of a primary carcinoma that are discontinuous from the primary and without histological evidence of residual lymph node or identifiable vascular or neural structures. If a vessel wall is identifiable on H&E, elastic or other stains, it should be classified as venous invasion (V1/2) or lymphatic invasion (L1). Similarly, if neural structures are identifiable, the lesion should be classified as perineural invasion (Pn1). The presence of tumour deposits does not change the primary tumour T category, but changes the node status (N) to pN1c if all regional lymph nodes are negative on pathological examination.

＊Source: TNM Classification of Malignant Tumours, Eighth edition, 2017, Wiley-Blackwell, Chichester UK.

Supplement 1-2 Carcinoma of the appendix
Appendix (ICD-O-3 C18.1)

T Primary Tumour

- TX   Primary tumour cannot be assessed
- T0   No evidence of primary tumour
- Tis   Carcinoma in situ: intraepithelial or invasion of lamina propria
- Tis (LAMN)   Low-grade appendiceal mucinous neoplasm confined to the appendix, (defined as involvement by acellular mucin or mucinous epithelium that may extend into muscularis propria)
- T1   Tumour invades submucosa
- T2   Tumour invades muscularis propria
- T3   Tumour invades subserosa or mesoappendix
- T4   Tumour perforates visceral peritoneum, including mucinous peritoneal tumours or acellular mucin on the serosa of the appendix or the mesoappendix and/or directly invades other organs or structures
  - T4a   Tumour perforates visceral peritoneum including mucinous peritoneal tumour or acellular mucin on the serosa of the appendix or mesoappendix
  - T4b   Tumour directly invades other organs or structures

N Regional Lymph Nodes

- NX   Regional Lymph Nodes cannot be assessed
- N0   No regional lymph node metastasis
- N1   Metastasis in 1 to 3 regional lymph nodes
  - N1a   Metastases in 1 regional lymph node
  - N1b   Metastases in 2–3 regional lymph nodes
  - N1c   Tumour deposit(s), i.e. satellites, in the subserosa or non-peritonealized pericolic or perirectal soft tissue, without regional lymph node metastasis
- N2   Metastasis in 4 or more regional lymph nodes

M Distant Metastasis

- M0   No distant metastasis
- M1   Distant metastasis
  - M1a   Intraperitoneal acellular mucin only
  - M1b   Intraperitoneal metastasis only, including mucinous epithelium
  - M1c   Non-peritoneal metastasis

G Histopathological Grading

GX Grade of differentiation cannot be assessed
G1 Well differentiated
G2 Moderately differentiated
G3 Poorly differentiated

Staging

Stage	T	N	M	G
Stage 0	Tis	N0	M0	
Stage 0	Tis (LAMN)	N0	M0	
Stage I	T1, T2	N0	M0	
Stage IIA	T3	N0	M0	
Stage IIB	T4a	N0	M0	
Stage IIC	T4b	N0	M0	
Stage IIIA	T1, T2	N1	M0	
Stage IIIB	T3, T4	N1	M0	
Stage IIIC	AnyT	N2	M0	
Stage IVA	AnyT	Any N	M1a	Any G
	AnyT	Any N	M1b	G1
Stage IVB	AnyT	Any N	M1b	G2, G3, GX
Stage IVC	AnyT	Any N	M1c	Any G

Table Stage of appendiceal cancer

M-Distant metastasis			M0			M1a	M1b	M1b	M1c
N-Regional lymph nodes / G-Tumour grade			N0	N1	N2	Any N or G	Any N / G1	Any N / G2/G3/GX	Any N or G
T-Primary tumour	Tis/Tis (LAMN)		0						
	T1		I	IIIA					
	T2				IIIC	IVA	IVB	IVC	
	T3		IIA	IIIB					
	T4a		IIB						
	T4b		IIC						

Source: TNM Classification of Malignant Tumours. Eighth Edition, 2017, Wiley-Blackwell, Chichester UK.

Supplement 1-3 Carcinoma of the anal canal
Anal Canal and Perianal Skin (ICD-O-3 C21, ICD-O-3 C44.5)

T Primary Tumour
TX	Primary tumour cannot be assessed
T0	No evidence of primary tumour
Tis	Carcinoma *in situ*, Bowen disease, high-grade squamous intraepithelial lesion (HSIL), anal intraepithelial neoplasia II–III (AIN II–III)
T1	Tumour 2 cm or less in greatest dimension
T2	Tumour more than 2 cm but not more than 5 cm in greatest dimension
T3	Tumour more than 5 cm in greatest dimension
T4	Tumour of any size invades adjacent organ (s), e.g., the vagina, urethra, bladder*

*Direct invasion of the rectal wall, perianal skin, subcutaneous tissue, or the sphincter muscle (s) alone not classified as T4.

N Regional Lymph Nodes
NX	Regional lymph nodes cannot be assessed
N0	No regional lymph node metastasis
N1	Metastasis in regional lymph node(s)
N1a	Metastases in inguinal, mesorectal, and/or internal iliac nodes
N1b	Metastases in external iliac nodes
N1c	Metastases in external iliac and in inguinal, mesorectal, and/or internal iliac nodes

M Distant Metastasis
M0	No distant metastasis
M1	Distant metastases

Stage

Stage	T	N	M
Stage 0	Tis	N0	M0
Stage I	T1	N0	M0
Stage IIA	T2	N0	M0
Stage IIB	T3	N0	M0
Stage IIIA	T1, T2	N1	M0
Stage IIIB	T4	N0	M0
Stage IIIC	T3, T4	N1	M0
Stage IV	Any T	Any N	M1

Table Stage of anal cancer

M-Distant metastasis		M0		M1
N-Regional lymph nodes		N0	N1	Any N
T-Primary tumour	Tis	0		IV
	T1	I	IIIA	
	T2	IIA		
	T3	IIB	IIIC	
	T4	IIIB		

Source: TNM Classification of Malignant Tumours. Eighth Edition, 2017, Wiley-Blackwell, Chichester UK.

Supplement 1-4 Well-differentiated neuroendocrine tumours (G1 and G2) of the colon and rectum, and the appendix

Colon and rectum

T Primary Tumour

TX   Primary tumour cannot be assessed
T0   No evidence of primary tumour
T1   Tumour invades lamina propria or submucosa or is no greater than 2 cm in size
    T1a   Tumour less than 1 cm in size
    T1b   Tumour between 1 or 2 cm in size
T2   Tumour invades muscularis propria or is greater than 2 cm in size
T3   Tumour invades subserosa, or non-peritonealized pericolic or perirectal tissues
T4   Tumour perforates the visceral peritoneum or invades other organs

N Regional Lymph Nodes

NX   Regional lymph nodes cannot be assessed
N0   No regional lymph node metastasis
N1   Regional lymph node metastasis

M Distant Metastasis

M0   No distant metastasis
M1   Distant metastasis
    M1a   Hepatic metastasis (is) only
    M1b   Extrahepatic metastasis (is) only
    M1c   Hepatic and extrahepatic metastases

Table   Stage of carcinoid of the colon and rectum

M-Distant metastasis		M0		M1
N-Regional lymph nodes		N0	N1	Any N
T-Primary tumor	T1	I	IIIB	IV
	T2	IIA		
	T3	IIB		
	T4	IIIA		

Source: TNM Classification of Malignant Tumours. Eighth Edition, 2017, Wiley-Blackwell, Chichester UK.

Appendix
T Primary Tumour
TX Primary tumour cannot be assessed
T0 No evidence of primary tumour
T1 Tumour 2 cm or less in greatest dimension
T2 Tumour more than 2 cm but not more than 4 cm in greatest dimension
T3 Tumour more than 4 cm or with subserosal invasion or involvement of the mesoappendix
T4 Tumour perforates peritoneum or invades other adjacent organs or structures, other than direct mural extension to adjacent subserosa, e.g., the abdominal wall and skeletal muscle

N Regional Lymph Nodes
NX Regional lymph nodes cannot be assessed
N0 No regional lymph node metastasis
N1 Regional lymph node metastasis

M Distant Metastasis
M0 No distant metastasis
M1 Distant metastasis
  M1a Hepatic metastasis (is) only
  M1b Extrahepatic metastasis (is) only
  M1c Hepatic and extrahepatic metastases

Table Stage of carcinoid of the appendix

M-Distant metastasis		M0		M1
N-Regional lymph nodes		N0	N1	Any N
T-Primary tumor	T1	I	III	IV
	T2	II		
	T3			
	T4			

Source: TNM Classification of Malignant Tumours. Eighth Edition, 2017, Wiley-Blackwell, Chichester UK.

Supplement 2 Summary of findings

【Preoperative clinical findings】
1. Preoperative CEA levels
2. Tumor location
3. Macroscopic types
4. cT (depth of tumor invasion)
5. cN (lymph node metastasis) Number of metastatic nodes
6. cM (distant metastasis) Metastasis site
7. cStage
8. Multiple colorectal cancers and multiple primary cancers

【Treatment】
9. Main treatment
10. Endoscopic/surgical treatments
    Endoscopic treatment method
    Surgical procedures
11. Extent of lymph node dissection (D), extent of lateral lymph node dissection (LD)
12. Organ of combined resection
13. Resected margin: PM DM RM HRM
14. Chemotherapy
15. Radiotherapy

【Pathological findings】
16. Tumor location
17. Macroscopic types
18. Tumor size
19. Proportion of the tumor in relation to the circumference of the bowel
20. Cancer involvement at resected margins
    Endoscopic resected specimen: HM VM
    Surgically resected specimen : PM DM RM HRM
21. pT (depth of tumor invasion)
    Submucosal invasion distance (T1 cancer only)
22. pN (lymph node metastasis and ND)
    Number of metastatic nodes/number of nodes retrieved
    Metastatic lymph nodes or ND(ND, ND(V+), ND(Pn+), ND(V&Pn+)) should be specified.

23. pM (only in case with histological diagnosis of distant metastasis)
24. Histological types
25. Infiltration pattern (INF)
26. Lymphovascular invasion (Ly, V)
27. Tumor budding (BD)
28. Perineural invasion (Pn)
29. pStage
30. Residual tumor
    Residual tumor following endoscopic treatment (ER)
    Residual tumor following surgical resection (R)
31. Curability with surgical treatment (Cur)
32. Assessment of response to chemotherapy and radiotherapy

Supplement 3 Checklist for pathological report

Item	Surgical treatments	Endoscopic treatments	refer
Procedure	Right hemicolectomy, Low anterior resection, etc.	Snare polypectomy, EMR, ESD	23-27
Tumor location	V, C, A, T, D, S, RS, Ra, Rb, P, (E)		7-10
Circumferential divisions of the wall of the rectum and anal canal	Ant, Post, Lt, Rt, Circ		
Macroscopic types	Type 0 [0-Ip, 0-Isp, 0-Is, 0-IIa, 0-IIb, 0-IIc, etc.], Type 1, Type 2, Type 3, Type 4, Type 5		10-11
Tumor size	Maximum diameter × maximum diameter in the orthogonal direction (mm)		10, 76-79
Proportion of the tumor in relation to the bowel circumferential	Percentage of the tumor maximum transverse diameter occupying the intestinal circumference (%)	—	10, 76-79
Histological type	pap, tub1, tub2, por1, por2, muc, sig, med, etc.		32-35, 62-74
Depth of tumor invasion*	pTX, pT0, pTis, pT1a, pT1b, pT2, pT3, pT4a, pT4b	pTX, pT0, pTis, pT1a, pT1b	12-13
	The depth of submucosal invasion is recorded (T1 cancer)		39-40
Infiltrative pattern	INFa, INFb, INFc		35
Lymphatic invasion	LyX, Ly0, Ly1[Ly1a, Ly1b, Ly1c]	LyX, Ly0, Ly1	35-36
Venous invasion	VX, V0, V1 [V1a, V1b, V1c], V2	VX, V0, V1, V2	36
Tumor budding	BDX, BD1, BD2, BD3		36-37
Perineural invasion	PnX, Pn0, Pn1a, Pn1b	—	37
Cancer involvement at resection margins	PMX, PM0, PM1; DMX, DM0, DM1; RMX, RM0, RM1; HRM0, HRM1	HMX, HM0, HM1; VMX, VM0, VM1	28-29
	In PM0/DM0/RM0, the margins of clearance are measured and recorded (mm)	In HM0/VM0, the margins of clearance are measured and recorded (mm)	
Lymph node metastasis*	pNX, pN0, pN1a, pN1b, pN2a, pN2b, pN3 The number of metastatic lymph nodes/The number of resected lymph nodes	—	17, 37-38
	The number of ND [ND, ND(V+), ND(Pn+), ND(V&Pn+)]		

Distant metastasis (when histological findings are available)	pM0, pM1a, pM1b, pM1c[M1c1, pM1c2]	—	17-20
	H, P, PUL, OSS, BRA, MAR, ADR etc.		
Liver metastasis	HX, H0, H1, H2, H3		
Peritoneal metastasis	PX, P0, P1, P2, P3		
Ascites cytology	Cy0, Cy1		
Pulmonary metastasis	PULX, PUL0, PUL1, PUL2		
pStage*	0, I, IIa, IIb, IIc, IIIa, IIIb, IIIc, IVa, IVb, IVc	—	20-21
Residual tumor	RX, R0, R1, R2	ERX, ER0, ER1a, ER1b, ER2	29-30
Curability following surgical resection	CurX, CurA, CurB, CurC	—	30
Histological assessment of response to chemotherapy and radiotherapy	Grade 0, Grade 1 [Grade 1a, Grade 1b], Grade 2, Grade 3		38-39

*If findings following preoperative treatment are documented, then prefix 'y' should be added (Pages 7, 22).

[**Example of documentation of findings**]

Surgical treatment: Sigmoidectomy, S, type 2, 60×40 mm, Proportion in relation to the bowel circumference 90% (45/50 mm), tub>muc, pT3, INFb, Ly1a, V1b, BD2, Pn1a, pPM0 (80 mm), pDM0 (40 mm), pRM0 (20 mm), pN2 (6/16) [ND 2, ND(V+) 1]*, pM1a (H1), pStage Iva, R0, CurB

*When out of 16 dissected lymph nodes, there are 3 metastatic lymph nodes, 2 ND, and 1 ND(V+)

[Documentation of ND]

e.g., When out of 11 dissected lymph nodes in the 251 area, there are 3 metastatic lymph nodes, 2 ND nodes, and 1 ND(Pn+)
#251: 6/11 [ND 2, ND(Pn+) 1]

Endoscopic resection: ESD, T, 0-IIa+IIc, 30×25 mm, tub1 with adenoma component, pT1a (SM, 380 μm), INFb, Ly0, V0, BD1, HM0 (3 mm, positive margin in adenoma components), VM0 (800 μm), ER0

Supplement 4 List of abbreviations

abbreviation	
A	ascending colon (p.7)
A	adventitia (p.12)
ADR	adrenals (p.18)
AI	direct invasion of other organs through the adventitia (p.12)
AN	autonomic nerve (p.27)
Ant	anterior (p.10)
BD	tumor budding (p.36)
BRA	brain (p.18)
C	cecum (p.7)
c	clinical findings (p.6)
Circ	circular (p.10)
CR	complete response (p.58)
Cur	curability, in surgical treatment (p.30)
Cy	cytology (p.19)
D	descending colon (p.7)
D	lymph node dissection (p.25)
DM	distal margin (p.29)
E	perianal skin (p.8)
EMR	endoscopic mucosal resection (p.23)
ER	residual tumor after endoscopic treatment (p.29)
ESD	endoscopic submucosal dissection (p.23)
EX	extramural cancer deposits without lymph node structure (p.37)
H	hepatic (metastasis) (p.18)
HM	horizontal margin (p.28)
H-N	hepatic node metastasis (p.19)
HRM	hepatic resection margin (p.29)
I	ileum (p.9)
INF	Infiltration pattern (p.35)
LD	lateral node dissection (p.26)
LST	laterally spreading tumor (p.11)
Lt	left (p.10)
Ly	lymphatic invasion (p.35)
LYM	lymph nodes (p.18)
M	mucosa (p.12)
M	distant metastasis (p.17)
MAR	bone marrow (p.18)
MP	muscularis propria (p.12)

continued

N	lymph node metastasis (p.17)	
ND	tumor nodule (p.37)	
ND(Pn+)	tumor nodule growing with perineural invasion (p.37)	
ND(V+)	tumor nodule growing with venous invasion (p.37)	
ND(V&Pn+)	tumor nodule growing with both venous and perineural invasion (p.37)	
NE	not evaluable (p.58)	
OSS	osseous (p.18)	
OTH	others (p.18)	
OVA	ovary (p.18)	
P	procto- (p.8)	
P	peritoneal metastasis (p.19)	
p	pathological findings (p.6)	
PM	proximal margin (p.29)	
Pn	perineural invasion (p.37)	
Post	posterior (p.10)	
PR	partial response (p.58)	
PS	performance status (p.31)	
PUL	pulmonary (metastasis) (p.19)	
r	recurrent (p.7)	
R	residual tumor after surgical treatment (p.29)	
Ra	upper rectum (above peritoneal reflection) (p.8)	
Rb	lower rectum (below peritoneal reflection) (p.8)	
RM	radial margin (p.29)	
RS	rectosigmoid (p.7)	
Rt	right (p.10)	
S	sigmoid colon (p.7)	
s	surgical findings (p.6)	
SE	serosa (p.12)	
SI	direct invasion of other organs through the serosa (p.12)	
SKI	skin (p.18)	
SM	submucosa (p.12)	
SS	subserosa (p.12)	
T	transverse colon (p.7)	
T	depth of tumor invasion (p.12)	
V	vermiform process (appendix) (p.8)	
V	venous invasion (p.36)	
VM	vertical margin (p.28)	
X	cannot be assessed (p.6)	
y	findings following preoperative treatment (p.7)	
yc	clinical findings following preoperative treatment (p.7)	
yp	pathological findings following preoperative treatment (p.7)	

Index

[A]

Abdominoperineal resection 24
Adenocarcinoma 32, 34, 35, 63, 71, 72
Adenocarcinoma associated with anal fistula 100
Adenoma 32, 34, 62
Adenosquamous carcinoma (asc) 33, 35, 64, 73, 94
adjuvant therapy 41
adverse events 59
Alive 42
Anal canal 8, 9, 34, 72
Anal verge 9
Anastomosis 26
Anastomotic recurrence 42
Anatomical anal canal 9
Anoderm 9
Ant 10
APC 23
Appendectomy 24
Ascending colon 7
autonomic nerves (AN) 27

[B]

B-cell lymphoma 33, 67
Benign epithelial neoplasia 34, 72
Benign epithelial tumor 32, 62, 71
Benign lymphoid polyp 33, 69
biopsy specimens 74
Bowen's disease 35
Burkitt's lymphoma 33, 68
Bypass surgery 25

[C]

Cancer involvement at resection margins 28
Cap polyposis 33, 69
Carcinoid tumor 33, 34, 35, 64, 65, 71, 73, 95

Carcinoma in situ 35
Cause of death 42
Cecum 7
Chemotherapy 31, 57
Clinical classifications (c) 20
Clinical findings (c) 6
Colostomy, ileostomy 25
Combined resection of adjacent organs and structures 27
Common Terminology Criteria for Adverse Events (CTCAE) 31, 59
Condyloma acuminatum 34, 100
Conjoined longitudinal muscle 9
Cowden syndrome, phosphate and tensin homolog (PTEN) hamartoma tumor syndrome 34
Cowden syndrome: PTEN hamartoma syndrome (Cowden polyp) 71
Cronkhite-Canada polyp 34, 70
Cronkhite-Canada syndrome 34, 70, 98
CTCAE 59
Curability (Cur) 30

[D]

Dead 42
Death due to colorectal cancer 42
Death due to other malignancy 42
Definition of endpoints and events 58
Dentate line 9
Depressed type 11
Depth of tumor invasion 12, 81
Descending colon 7
diagnostic imaging findings 6

Diffuse large B-cell lymphoma 33, 68
Diffusely infiltrating type 10
disease-free survival (DFS) 58
Distal margin (DM) 29
Distant metastasis (M) 17
Downward lymph nodes 45

[E]

efficacy endpoints 58
Elastica van Gieson staining 36
Elevated type 11
Endocrine cell carcinoma 33, 35, 65, 73, 95
Endometriosis 34, 69
Endoscopic mucosal resection (EMR) 23
Endoscopic submucosal dissection (ESD) 23
Endoscopic treatment 23
Evaluation of resected specimens 32
EX 38, 83
Exploratory laparotomy 25
Extent of lateral lymph node dissection (LD) 26
Extent of lymph node dissection (D) 25
Extent of primary tumor (T) 13
External anal sphincter (Deep)/(Superficial)/(Subcutaneous) 9
Extramammary Paget disease 101
Extramammary Paget's disease 35, 73
Extramucosal (fistula-associated, perianal) adenocarcinoma 35
Extramural cancer deposits without lymph node structure (EX) 37, 83
extramural discontinuous cancer

spread (EX) 1
Extramural (perianal) adenocarcinoma 72

[F]

Familial adenomatous polyposis (FAP) 22, 23, 34, 70
Family history and hereditary diseases 22
Flat type 11
Follicular lymphoma 33, 67

[G]

Gastrointestinal stromal tumors (GISTs) 67
GIST (Gastrointestinal stromal tumor) 33
Goblet cell carcinoid 34, 71, 99
Grade 38
Grade classification for patients with pulmonary metastasis 20
Grade of patients with liver metastasis 18
Group classification 39, 74

[H]

Hamartomatous polyp 33, 69
Handling of biopsy materials 76
Handling of endoscopically resected specimens 79
Handling of resected specimens 76
handling of surgically resected specimens 76
Hartmann procedure 24
Hematogenous metastasis 43
hereditary non-polyposis colorectal cancer (HNPCC) 23
Hereditary tumors and gastrointestinal polyposis 34, 70
Hidradenoma papilliferum 34
High anterior resection 24
High-grade intraepithelial neoplasia 34
Histological assessment of biopsy specimens 39, 74
Histological criteria for the assessment of response to chemotherapy/radiotherapy 38
Histological types 62
Hodgkin lymphoma 68
Hodgkin's lymphoma 33
Horizontal margin 28
Hyperplastic (metaplastic) polyp 33, 68, 96
Hyperplastic nodule 33, 68, 96
Hypogastric nerve 27

[I]

Ileocecal resection 24
ileocecal valve 8
Iliac artery 44
Inferior mesenteric artery 15, 44
Infiltration pattern (INF) 35
Inflammatory fibroid polyp 33, 69
Inflammatory myoglandular polyp 33, 69
Inflammatory polyp and polyposis 33, 69
intermediate lymph nodes 14, 15, 44
Intermuscular groove 9
Internal anal sphincter 9
International Collaborative Group on Hereditary Non-Polyposis Colorectal Cancer (ICG-HNPCC) 23
Intersphincteric resection 24

[J]

JCCRC 1
Juvenile polyp 33, 68, 97
Juvenile polyposis 34, 70

[L]

lateral lymph node dissection (LD) 26
lateral lymph nodes 14, 45
laterally spreading tumor (LST) subtype 53, 54, 55
Laterally spreading tumors (LSTs) 11
Left hemicolectomy 24
Lipoma and lipomatosis 33, 67
Liver metastasis (H) 18, 43
Local excision 24
Local recurrence 42
Low anterior resection 24
Lower rectum 8
Low-grade appendiceal mucinous neoplasm 34, 71, 99
Low-grade intraepithelial neoplasia 34
Lt 10
Lumbar splanchnic nerve 27
Lung metastasis 43
Lymph node dissection 25
Lymph node groups 13, 44, 46
Lymph node metastasis (N) 17, 43
Lymph node station number 13
lymph node structure 83
Lymph nodes proximal to the main lymph nodes 45
Lymphatic invasion (Ly) 35, 82
Lymphoma 33, 67
Lymphovascular invasion 35
Lynch syndrome 23, 34, 70
Lynch syndrome (hereditary non-polyposis colorectal cancer) 22

[M]

Macroscopic examination 76
main lymph nodes 14, 15, 44
Malignant epithelial neoplasia 34, 71
Malignant epithelial tumors 32, 35, 63, 72
Malignant lymphoma 34, 35, 71, 74
Malignant melanoma 35, 73, 101
MALT lymphoma 67
Mantle cell lymphoma 33, 67
Measurement of submucosal invasion distance 56
Measurement of the depth of invasion 39
Measurement of the depth of invasion in T1 cancers 40

Medullary carcinoma (med)   32, 64, 94
Mesenchymal neoplasia   35
Mesenchymal tumor   34, 74
metachronous   23
metastasis   42
Metastatic tumors   33, 68
Miscellaneous histological types of epithelial malignant tumors   66
Miscellaneous tumor   33, 67
Moderately differentiated tubular adenocarcinoma (tub2)   91
Moderately differentiated type (tub2)   32, 63
Mucinous adenocarcinoma (muc)   32, 64
Mucinous carcinoma (muc)   93
Mucosa-associated lymphoid tissue (MALT) lymphoma   33
Mucosal prolapse syndrome   33, 69
Multiple colorectal cancers   22, 41
multiple primary cancers   22, 41
Myogenic tumor   33
Myogenic tumors   66

[N]
ND   37, 38, 83
Neurogenic tumor   33, 67
Non-epithelial tumor   33, 67, 71, 74
Non-solid type (por2)   32, 63, 92

[O]
Obturator nerves   46
Other lymph nodes   45
Other lymphomas   68
Other palliative procedures   25
Other types of colectomy   24
Overall survival (OS)   58

[P]
Papillary adenocarcinoma (pap)   32, 63, 89
Partial colectomy   24
pathological classifications (p)   20
Pathological findings (p)   6
Pedunculated type   11
Pelvic nerve plexus   46
pelvic plexus   27
performance status (PS)   31
Perianal skin (E)   8, 9
pericolic lymph nodes   14
pericolic/perirectal lymph nodes   15, 44
Perineural invasion (Pn)   37, 84, 85
Peritoneal metastasis (P)   19, 43
Peutz-Jeghers syndrome   34, 70, 98
physical findings   6
Polypectomy   24
Polypoid type   10
Poorly differentiated adenocarcinoma (por)   32, 63
Poorly differentiated adenocarcinoma: non-solid type (por2)   92
Poorly differentiated adenocarcinoma: solid type (por1)   92
Post   10
Proctocolectomy   24
progression-free survival (PFS)   58
Protruded type   11
Proximal margin (PM)   29
Pseudoinvasion of adenoma   88
pseudopeduncle   50
Puborectal muscle   9
Pulmonary metastasis (PUL)   19

[R]
r   7
Radial margin (circumferential resection margin) (RM)   29
Radiotherapy   31, 57
RECIST   58
Rectal mucosa   9
Rectal-type adenocarcinoma   35, 72
Rectosigmoid   7
Recurrence   42

Recurrence in regional lymph nodes   42
Regional lymph nodes   14, 15
relapse-free survival (RFS)   58
Resection rate   41
Residual tumor following endoscopic treatment (ER)   29
Residual tumor following surgical treatment (R)   29
Response Evaluation Criteria in Solid Tumors (RECIST)   31, 58
Right hemicolectomy   24
Rt   10

[S]
Serrated adenoma   88
Serrated lesion   34
Serrated polyposis/hyperplastic polyposis   34, 70
Sessile serrated adenoma/polyp (SSA/P)   33, 68, 97
Sessile type   11
Sigmoid colon   7
Sigmoidectomy   24
Signet-ring cell carcinoma (sig)   32, 64, 93
Snare polypectomy   23
Solid type (por1)   32, 63, 92
Squamous cell carcinoma (scc)   33, 35, 64, 73
Squamous cell papilloma   34
Squamous intraepithelial neoplasia   34, 72
Stage grouping   20
Stage grouping of the TNM classification   22
station number   13, 44, 46
Subpedunculated type   11
Subtotal colectomy   24
Subtypes of macroscopic type 0   50, 51, 52
Superficial type   10, 11
Superior border of puborectal sling   9
Superior hypogastric plexus   27
Superior mesenteric artery   15, 44

Surgical findings (s) 6
Survival analysis 42
synchronous 23
Synchronous and metachronous tumors 23

[T]

T-cell lymphoma 33, 68
time to treatment failure (TTF) 58
Total colectomy 24
Total pelvic exenteration 24
Traditional serrated adenoma 32, 62
Transitional epithelium 9
Transverse colon 7
Treatment-related death 42
Tubular adenocarcinoma (tub) 32, 63
Tubular adenoma 32, 62, 85, 86
Tubulovillous adenoma 32, 62, 87
Tumor budding (BD) 36, 83
Tumor location 7
Tumor-like lesion 35, 74
Tumor-like lesions 33, 34, 68, 71

[U]

Ulcerated type with clear margin 10
Ulcerated type with infiltration 10
Ultra-low anterior resection 24
Unclassifiable tumors 68
Unclassified type 11
Upper rectum 8

[V]

Vascular tumor 33, 67
vascular/perineural invasion 17, 37, 83
Venous invasion (V) 36, 82
Vermiform appendix 8, 34, 71
Vertical margin (VM) 28
Victoria blue staining 36
Vienna classification 76
Villous adenoma 32, 62, 87

[W]

Well differentiated tubular adenocarcinoma (tub1) 89, 90
Well differentiated type (tub1) 32, 63
WHO classification 65, 66

[Y]

y 7, 22
yc 7, 22
yp 7, 22

大腸癌取扱い規約（英語版第 3 版）
定価(本体 4,200 円＋税)

1997 年 10 月 20 日　英語版第 1 版発行
2009 年 1 月 13 日　英語版第 2 版発行
2019 年 4 月 25 日　英語版第 3 版第 1 刷発行

編　者　　大腸癌研究会

発行者　　福村　直樹

発行所　　金原出版株式会社
　　　　　〒113-0034 東京都文京区湯島 2-31-14
　　　　　電話　編集　(03)3811-7162
　　　　　　　　営業　(03)3811-7184
　　　　　FAX　　　　(03)3813-0288　　　Ⓒ 大腸癌研究会, 1997, 2019
　　　　　振替口座　00120-4-151494　　　　　　検印省略
　　　　　http://www.kanehara-shuppan.co.jp/　　Printed in Japan

Japanese Classification of Colorectal, Appendiceal, and Anal Carcinoma
Third English Edition

Japanese Society for Cancer of the Colon and Rectum

ISBN 978-4-307-20395-1　　　　印刷・製本／三報社印刷㈱

JCOPY ＜出版者著作権管理機構　委託出版物＞

本書の無断複製は著作権法上での例外を除き禁じられています。複製される場合は，
そのつど事前に，出版者著作権管理機構（電話 03-5244-5088, FAX 03-5244-5089,
e-mail : info@jcopy.or.jp）の許諾を得てください。

小社は捺印または貼付紙をもって定価を変更致しません。
乱丁，落丁のものはお買上げ書店または小社にてお取り替え致します。